Lecture Notes on Endocrinology

WILLIAM JEFFCOATE
MB BChir FRCP
Consultant Physician, City Hospital, Nottingham

FIFTH EDITION

OXFORD

BLACKWELL SCIENTIFIC PUBLICATIONS

LONDON EDINBURGH BOSTON

MELBOURNE PARIS BERLIN VIENNA

© 1967, 1978, 1982, 1987, 1993,
Blackwell Scientific Publications
Editorial Offices:
Osney Mead, Oxford OX2 0EL
25 John Street, London, WC1N 2BL
23 Ainslie Place, Edinburgh EH3 6AJ
238 Main Street, Cambridge
    Massachusetts 02142, USA
54 University Street, Carlton
    Victoria 3053, Australia

Other Editorial Offices:
Librairie Arnette SA
2, rue Casimir-Delavigne
75006 Paris
France

Blackwell Wissenschafts-Verlag
Meinekestrasse 4
D-1000 Berlin 15
Germany

Blackwell MZV
Feldgasse 13
A-1238 Wien
Austria

First published 1967
Second edition 1978
Reprinted 1979
Third edition 1982
Fourth edition 1987
Fifth edition 1993
Four Dragons edition 1993

Set by Semantic Graphics, Singapore
Printed and bound in Great Britain by
Hartnolls Ltd, Bodmin, Cornwall

DISTRIBUTORS

Marston Book Services Ltd
PO Box 87
Oxford OX2 0DT
(*Orders*: Tel: 0865 791155
            Fax: 0865 791927
            Telex: 837515)

USA
Blackwell Scientific Publications, Inc.
238 Main Street
Cambridge, MA 02142
(*Orders*: Tel: 800 759–6102
                617 876–7000)

Canada
Times Mirror Professional Publishing, Ltd
130 Flaska Drive
Markham, Ontario L6G 1B8
(*Orders*: Tel: 800 268–4178
                416 470–6739)

Australia
Blackwell Scientific Publications Pty Ltd
54 University Street,
Carlton, Victoria 3053
(*Orders*: Tel: 03 347–5552)

A catalogue record for this title
is available from the British Library

ISBN 0-632-03348-7
ISBN 0-632-03535-8 (Four Dragons)

Library of Congress
Cataloging in Publication Data

Jeffcoate, William.
    Lecture notes on endocrinology /
    William Jeffcoate. — 5th ed.
        p.   cm.
    Rev ed. of: Lecture notes on endocrinology /
    Ronald F. Fletcher. — 4th ed. 1987
    Includes bibliographical references and index.
    ISBN 0-632-03348-7
    1. Endocrine glands — Diseases.
    2. Endocrinology.
        I. Fletcher, Ronald F.   Lecture notes on
    endocrinology.   II. Title.
    [DNLM: 1. Endocrine Diseases.
    WK 100 J45L]
    RC648.J44 1993
    616.4—dc20
    DNLM/DLC

Contents

Preface, vi

List of Abbreviations, viii

1   The Endocrine System, 1

2   The Hypothalamus and Pituitary, 25

3   The Thyroid Gland, 60

4   The Adrenal Gland and the Kidney, 79

5   Endocrinological Aspects of Malignancy, 107

6   Gut Hormones — Hormones of the Enteroinsular Axis, 109

7   The Thymus, 120

8   Diabetes Mellitus, 121

9   Fat and Fat Metabolism, 151

10 Differentiation, Growth and Development, 173

11 Male Sexual Function — Andrology, 193

12 Female Sexual Function — Gynaecological Endocrinology, 204

13 Calcium Metabolism and Disorders of Bone, 219

Index, 234

Preface

While the clinical practice of endocrinology is largely concerned with diseases of endocrine glands, the science of endocrinology is more far-reaching. It concerns the study of hormones, with the word hormone being applied to any chemical which mediates communication between cells. There is great overlap with neuro-pharmacology, and there will be ever-increasing overlap with molecular biology as more details of intracellular processes are unravelled. It is for reasons such as these that any writer of a textbook of endocrinology has to think hard about what to include, and what to omit. This is especially true of a book which is designed for the undergraduate and the general clinician who perhaps wish to learn only the basic essentials.

This edition of *Lecture Notes on Endocrinology* is entirely new. An attempt is made in each section to review both the physiology of hormones, and the basic principles of the pathology, diagnosis and management of endocrine diseases. As always in this field, it is inevitable that rather rare diseases seem to occupy inappropriate space, whereas common ones are crowded. However, emphasis has been placed on those disorders which most commonly concern general clinicians, such as thyroid diseases and hirsutism. Subjects which may be considered as only vaguely 'endocrinological' — obesity, lipids and atherogenesis, impotence and disorders of bone — are also included.

Perhaps the greatest dilemma facing any author of an endocrinology textbook of this size is whether or not to include diabetes and if so, how much? The answer is that diabetes must always be included, because it is the commonest of all endocrine diseases, even though different people will have different ideas of the amount of space to be devoted to it. It is a disease which affects all organs and tissues of the body, and it is one which requires very special skills in management. If it is to be covered at all, it has to be covered in some detail. With these thoughts in mind I have included what I think is necessary for a general practitioner (with the words being used in the widest sense) to know, but have deliberately avoided attempting to write an authoritative review.

I have included no references, because anyone who is at all interested in a subject should easily be able to find their own. Furthermore, I believe that references in a textbook of this kind can sometimes be unhelpful. They will be selected according to an author's bias, and may perhaps be used to give authenticity to his or her belief. I have preferred to state my opinion, unsupported, and have not hesitated to disagree with what I regard as ill-substantiated dogma. I hope that some will disagree with me.

In completing this text, I am deeply indebted to many people. Those with whom I worked in training: Roger Short, John Nabarro, Michael Besser and Lesley Rees, and the many with whom I have worked in Nottingham. Of these I am especially grateful to Geoff Bennett, Fiona Broughton-Pipkin, Rex Coupland, Julian Davis, Tim Dornan, Ian Fellows, Nick Galloway, Sheila Gardiner, Simon Heller, David Hosking, Derek Johnston, Ron Jones, Nadina Lincoln, Richard Long, Christine Marenah, Shaughan O'Brien, Donal O'Donoghue, Ian Peacock, Colin Selby, Dennis Shale, Mike Sokal, Dave White and Malcolm Wilson. In acknowledging their help, I would be the last to suggest that they should be held accountable for opinions which I have expressed.

William Jeffcoate

List of Abbreviations

AII	angiotensin II
ACE	angiotensin converting enzyme
ACTH	adrenocorticotrophic hormone
ADH	antidiuretic hormone
AID/AIH	artificial insemination using semen from donor/husband
AMH	antimullerian hormone
AMP	adenosine monophosphate
ANF	atrial natriuretic factor, atriopeptin
Apo	apoprotein
ATP	adenosine triphosphate
ATPase	adenosine triphosphatase
AVP	arginine vasopressin
BAT	brown adipose tissue
BMR	basal metabolic rate
C-cells	parafollicular cells of the thyroid
C-peptide	connecting peptide of pro-insulin
CAH	congenital adrenal hyperplasia
cAMP	cyclic AMP
CAPD	chronic ambulatory peritoneal dialysis
CBG	cortisol-binding globulin
CCF	congestive cardiac failure
CCK	cholecystokinin
cGMP	cyclic guanosine monophosphate
CGRP	calcitonin gene-related peptide
CJD	Creutzfeld–Jakob disease
CLIP	corticotrophin-like intermediate lobe peptide
COMT	catechol-O-methyl transferase
CRF	corticotrophin-releasing factor
CRH	corticotrophin-releasing hormone
CSF	cerebrospinal fluid
CT	computed tomography
Da	Daltons
DBP	vitamin D-binding protein
DCT	distal convoluted tubule
DDAVP	deamino-D-arginine vasopressin
DG	diacylglycerol
DHEA	dehydroepiandrosterone
DHEAS	dehydroepiandrosterone sulphate
DHT	dihydrotestosterone

DI	diabetes insipidus
DIDMOAD	diabetes insipidus, diabetes mellitus, optic atrophy, deafness
DIT	diiodotyrosine
DKA	diabetic ketoacidosis
DM	diabetes mellitus
DNA	deoxyribonucleic acid
DOPA	dihydroxyphenylalanine
DVLC/DVLA	Driver and Vehicle Licensing Centre/Authority
ECF	extracellular fluid
ECG	electrocardiogram
EEG	electroencephalogram
EPO	erythropoietin
ESR	erythrocyte sedimentation rate
FFAs	free fatty acids
FH	familial hypercholesterolaemia
FSH	follicle-stimulating hormone
GFR	glomerular filtration rate
GH	growth hormone
GHRH/GRH	growth hormone-releasing hormone
GHRIH	growth hormone-release-inhibiting hormone, somatostatin
GIFT	gamete intraFallopian transfer
GIP	glucose-dependent insulinotropic peptide, gastric inhibitory peptide
GnRH	gonadotrophin-releasing hormone, also called LHRH
GP	general practitioner
GRH	growth hormone-releasing hormone, also called GHRH
GTP	guanosine triphosphate
GTPase	guanosine triphosphatase
HAM	hypoparathyroidism, Addison's disease, moniliasis
hCG	human chorionic gonadotrophin
HDL	high density lipoprotein
hGH	biosynthetic growth hormone
5HIAA	5-hydroxyindole acetic acid
hnRNA	heterogeneous nuclear ribonucleic acid
HONK	hyperosmolar non-ketotic diabetic coma
HPL	human placental lactogen
HRT	hormone replacement therapy
HSL	hormone sensitive lipase
5-HT	5-hydroxytryptamine
IAPP	islet amyloid polypeptide, amylin
ICA	islet cell antibodies
IDL	intermediate density lipoprotein, VLDL remnant
IGF	insulin-like growth factor
IGF-BPs	IGF binding proteins, also called SBPs
IGT	impaired glucose tolerence
ILs	interleukins

INFs	interferons
IP_3	inositol triphosphate
ITT	insulin tolerence, or hypoglycaemia stress, test
IVF	*in vitro* fertilization
LCAT	lecithin–cholesterol acyltransferase
LDL	low density lipoprotein
LFTs	liver function tests
LH	luteinizing hormone
LHRH	luteinizing hormone-releasing hormone
β-LPH	β-lipotrophin
LPL	lipoprotein lipase
MAO	monoamine oxidase
MBq	megabecquerels
MEN	multiple endocrine neoplasia
MHC	major histocompatibility gene
MIBG	metaiodobenzylguanidine
MIF	Mullerian inhibitory factor
MIT	monoiodotyrosine
MODY	maturity onset diabetes of young people
MRI	magnetic resonance imaging
mRNA	messenger RNA
MSH	melanocyte-stimulating hormone
NEFAs	non-esterified fatty acids
NPY	neuropeptide Y
NSAIDs	non-steroidal anti-inflammatory agents
OAF	osteoclast-activating factors
1,25-OHCC	1,25-dihydroxy vitamin D
24,25-OHCC	24,25-dihydroxy vitamin D
25-OHCC	25-hydroxy vitamin D
opDDD	ortho, para-DDD, mitotane
PCO	polycystic ovary (disease/syndrome)
PCT	post-coital test
PDGF	platelet-derived growth factor
PGF/PGE/PGA	prostaglandin F/E/A
PGI_2	prostacyclin
PI	phosphatidyl inositol
POMC	pro-opiomelanocortin
PP	pancreatic polypeptide
PPPT	painless post-partum thyroiditis
PTH	parathyroid hormone
PTHrp	parathyroid hormone-related protein
PTU	propylthiouracil
RBF	renal blood flow
RNA	ribonucleic acid
rT_3	reverse (inactive) T_3
SBPs	somatomedin binding proteins, also called IGF-BPs

SHBG	sex-hormone binding globulin
SIADH	syndrome of inappropriate antidiuretic hormone secretion
T_4	thyroxine
T_3	triiodothyronine
TBG	thyroxine binding protein
TFT	thyroid function tests
TIA	transient ischaemic attack
TNF	tumour necrosis factor
TRH	thyrotrophin-releasing hormone
tRNA	transfer RNA
TSH	thyroid-stimulating hormone, thyrotrophin
TSI	thyroid stimulating immunoglobulins (previously called LATS-P)
TXA_2	thromboxane
UV	ultraviolet
VIP	vasoactive intestinal polypeptide
Vitamin D_2	ergocalciferol
Vitamin D_3	cholecalciferol
VLDL	very low density lipoprotein
VMA	vanillyl mandelic acid
VNM	ventromedial nucleus (of the hypothalamus)

Chapter 1
The Endocrine System

INTRODUCTION

Hormones are molecules which are released by one cell to act on another which may be close by or distant: they are chemical messengers. They represent one way in which cells communicate with each other.

A hormone may be transported by the blood stream, or other body fluid, or it may diffuse locally to act on adjacent cells. Blood-borne hormones are called 'endocrine'. Hormones which act on adjacent cells are called 'paracrine'. Hormones can also feed back to act on the cell which releases them, and these are called 'autocrine'.

Hormones are phylogenetically ancient, and the same chemicals which communicate between the cells of humans can be found in the cells of fish, insects, plants and even unicellular organisms.

There are five broad chemical classes of hormone:
1 Proteins and polypeptides.
2 Monoamines: derivatives of phenylalanine and tryptophan.
3 Iodothyronines.
4 Cholesterol derivatives and steroids.
5 Arachidonic acid derivatives.

The protein/polypeptide group is the largest and most diverse. The nature of peptide synthesis has allowed the evolution of a vast range of hormones by mutation. Different species, and different classes and orders of organism tend to have evolved their own specific form of peptide hormone, as well as of each hormone receptor.

In contrast, the number of different hormones in the non-peptide groups is small, and they tend to be structurally identical in different species.

HORMONE TYPES

Protein and polypeptide hormones

Synthesis

The nucleotide sequence of deoxyribonucleic acid (DNA) is transcribed by ribonucleic acid (RNA) polymerases to the complementary sequence of heterogeneous nuclear RNA (hnRNA) (see Fig. 1.1). Heterogeneous nuclear RNA is converted to messenger RNA (mRNA) by the removal of non-translated base sequences (introns). Messenger RNA leaves the nucleus and associates with the ribosomes of the endoplasmic reticulum. Ribosomes contribute to the configurational changes within the assembling polypeptide. The cluster of ribosomes around any one mRNA sequence is called a polyribosome. The base sequence of

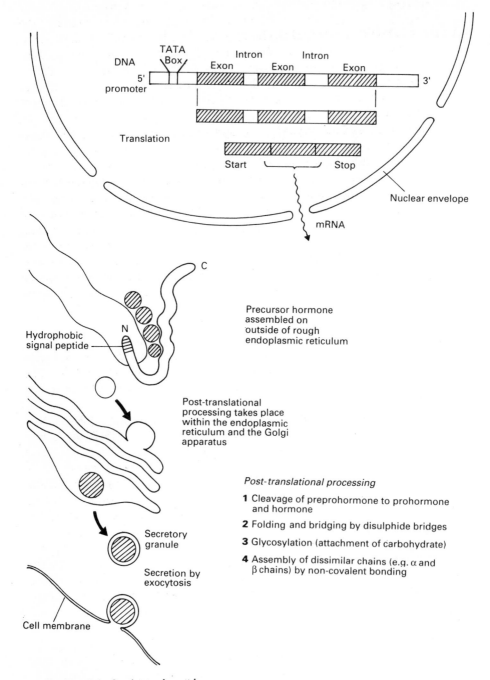

Fig. 1.1. Synthesis of peptides.

the ribosome-bound RNA is translated into a polypeptide with each triplet of bases (codon) signalling the attachment of a certain amino acid. The amino acids are transported to the polyribosome by transfer RNA (tRNA), to which each is attached via an identical three-base sequence (anticodon). A total of 64 possible codons can be derived from combinations of the four nucleotides — adenine, guanine, thymine and cytosine. Three are used as signal codons to initiate or terminate translation, and the remaining 61 are used to code for the 20 amino acids. The codon sequence of mRNA is translated progressively from the 5′ to the 3′ terminal, and the polypeptide is constructed progressively from the carboxy (C-) to the amino (N-) terminal.

The polypeptide is assembled on the cytoplasmic surface of the endoplasmic reticulum, but is transferred to the non-cytoplasmic surface for co-translational and post-translational processing. This transfer is achieved by the addition of a hydrophobic signal peptide sequence to its N-terminal. The peptide draws the polypeptide protein sequence through the membrane into the Golgi lumen. With the signal peptide still attached the peptide is known as a preprohormone. After co-translational cleavage, it is called a prohormone. Further post-translational processing, including cleavage and/or glycosylation by addition of carbohydrate moieties, results in mature hormone being packed in secretory granules, ready for release by exocytosis.

Secondary structure

Most peptide hormones are single-chain polypeptides, either straight or looped into a ring. Insulin is looped into a ring before having the end of the loop (the 'connecting' or C-peptide) cleaved, leaving two chains linked by disulphide bridges (Fig. 1.2).

The glycoprotein family of hormones (luteinizing hormone (LH), follicle-stimulating hormone (FSH), thyroid-stimulating hormone (TSH) and human chorionic gonadotrophin (hCG)) each have two chains, with two dissimilar α and β chains linked non-covalently (see Fig. 1.3). The α subunit of 92 amino acids is the same in all four hormones. The β subunit of 118 amino acids is variable, although there are some sequence homologies because the four hormones are related phylogenetically. The variable region of the β chain allows interaction with specific receptors, while the sequence homologies in the β subunit ensure binding to the α subunit. The ability to activate adenylate cyclase in the target tissue is shared by the four hormones and is dependent on the common α subunit. The variations in the β chain do not result in absolute specificity of action: when hCG levels are very high, as in chorioncarcinoma, the hCG can cause thyrotoxicosis by stimulating the TSH receptor.

Secretion

Peptide hormones are usually released in bursts, which may be in response to an unprogrammed stimulus (e.g. adrenocorticotrophic hormone (ACTH) release in response to physical trauma) or may be regular and pulsatile (e.g. the regular 13-minute cycling of insulin release or the rather less regular 90-minute pulses of LH release). Hormones such as growth hormone (GH) and prolactin have a basic

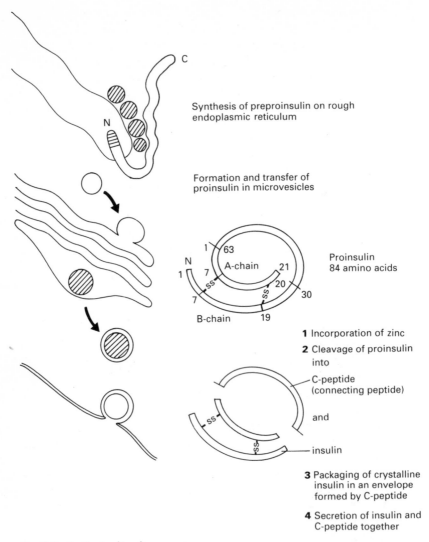

C

N

Synthesis of preproinsulin on rough
endoplasmic reticulum

Formation and transfer of
proinsulin in microvesicles

1   63
N   A-chain   21
1   7   20
ss   ss   30
7
B-chain   19

Proinsulin
84 amino acids

1 Incorporation of zinc

2 Cleavage of proinsulin
into

C-peptide
(connecting peptide)

and

insulin

3 Packaging of crystalline
insulin in an envelope
formed by C-peptide

4 Secretion of insulin and
C-peptide together

Fig. 1.2. Synthesis of insulin.

tonic level of release, with superadded bursts. The burst of hormone may have a
qualitatively, as well as a quantitatively, different action. Peptide hormones tend to
be stored in secretory granules in the cytoplasm, so that they can be released
rapidly when required. Catecholamines are also stored in this way, but hormones
which are released more slowly, such as thyroid hormones and steroids, are not.

When hormones are released in pulses or bursts, the body needs a rapid
mechanism for their inactivation and clearance. Such rapid metabolism is a
feature of many peptide hormones, as well as catecholamines, and they may have
an effective plasma half-life of only seconds or minutes. This contrasts with
steroids and thyroid hormones which have a longer half-life of disappearance.

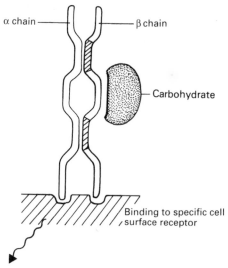

α chain

β chain

Carbohydrate

Binding to specific cell
surface receptor

Binding to α-chain
receptor activates
adenylate cyclase

Fig. 1.3. Structure of glycoprotein hormones. The four glycoprotein hormones (luteinizing hormone, LH; follicle-stimulating hormone, FSH; thyroid-stimulating hormone, TSH; human chorionic gonadotrophin, hCG) have identical α chains. The β chains differ but have some shared sequences (shaded) to ensure binding to the α chains. Binding to the specific cell surface β receptor allows the α chain to activate adenylate cyclase.

Transport

Peptides are water-soluble and mostly circulate freely in plasma. They do not need binding to carrier substances to be transported to target organs (even though one or two, e.g. GH, do actually have binding proteins). At the target site they associate with cell-surface receptors. These receptors are glycoproteins of varying size: from 300 to 360 000 Da. Receptors are not stable, fixed structures — they are constantly altering, being made available or not available, and even moving across the surface of the cell.

Target cell interaction

It has been demonstrated that insulin receptors move when activated by insulin binding to them. The hormone–receptor complex migrates across the cell surface to specific areas, called coated pit regions, where endocytosis takes place (see Fig. 1.4). The complex stays packeted in a fold of cell membrane and enters the cell. The packet is called the endosome. Within the endosome the receptor and hormone dissociate, partly in response to reduced pH. The hormone then initiates a response by a second messenger, intracellular system, while the receptor is recycled to the cell surface.

Down-regulation

Peptide hormones control the number of cell-surface receptors which are

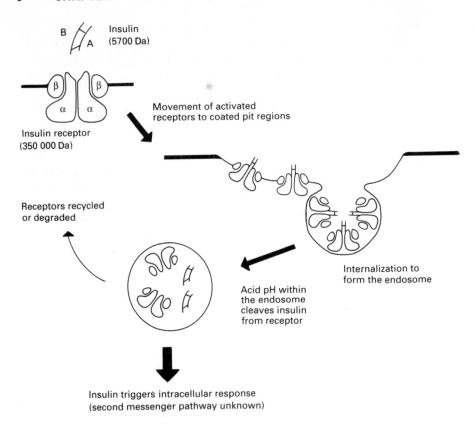

Fig. 1.4. Interaction of insulin with its cell-surface receptor.

expressed. If peptides are secreted in excess, the number of receptors is reduced — 'receptor down-regulation'.

Clearance

Peptide which is taken into the target cell is broken down *in situ*. Circulating peptide is cleared or inactivated by circulating or tissue-bound peptidases. These may be exopeptidases, which cleave terminal amino acids from the chain, or endopeptidases which split the chain in the middle. In general, peptides which are cleared or inactivated more rapidly (e.g. ACTH or enkephalins), are broken down by circulating enzymes, whereas those with a rather longer half-life (e.g. prolactin, insulin) are metabolized by tissue-bound enzymes — particularly those in the kidney and in the liver and lung.

Monoamines

Derivatives of phenylalanine

There are three phenylalanine derivatives which act either as hormones or neurotransmitters: noradrenaline, adrenaline and dopamine, and all are widely distributed through the body. All three are secreted as true hormones by the adrenal medulla, but it is not known how their separate actions are integrated, nor how their release by the adrenal medulla is integrated with release by sympathetic nerve terminals. No special harm seems to result from removal of the adrenal medulla.

Adrenaline and noradrenaline are catecholamines: the term 'catechol' indicates the presence of the two hydroxyl groups on the benzene ring.

Synthesis

The rate-limiting step in the biosynthesis of adrenaline and noradrenaline in the adrenal medulla is the initial conversion of tyrosine to dihydroxyphenylalanine (DOPA) by tyrosine hydroxylase (see Fig. 1.5). The 'nor' of noradrenaline indicates that the 'N' is 'or' ('*ohne Radikal*', i.e. without its methyl group). Methylation of adrenaline is catalysed by phenylethanolamine-*N*-methyltransferase. This enzyme is potentiated by glucocorticoids (cortisol). This action of cortisol

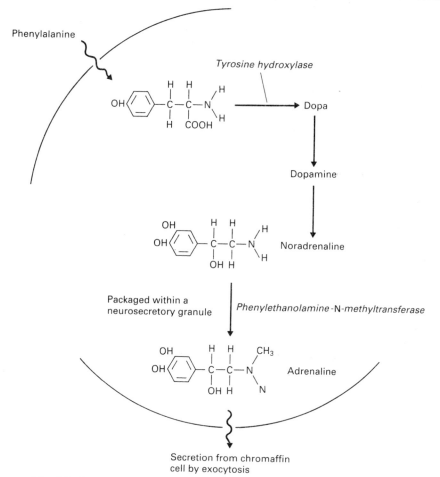

Fig. 1.5. Synthesis of catecholamines.

indicates how the adrenal cortex may modify the function of the adrenal medulla, and may be one reason why the two glands are closely related anatomically, even though they are embryologically distinct.

The amines are stored in secretory granules in the adrenal medulla. Those containing adrenaline are more numerous, and are larger. Other substances, including peptide hormones such as enkephalins and somatostatin, are also present in these secretory granules.

Secretion

Amines are released from the adrenal medulla in response to either a nervous (preganglionic sympathetic fibres innervate the gland) or a humoral stimulus, e.g. nicotine and tyrosine. Release is pulsatile; inactivation and clearance are rapid. Amines are water-soluble and are not bound to carrier proteins in the blood.

Target-cell interaction

The amines interact with families of related cell-surface receptors: α_1 and α_2, β_1 and β_2 receptors for catecholamines, D_1 and D_2 receptors for dopamine. The activated receptor induces a cellular response by generating cyclic adenosine monophoshate (cAMP). The results of receptor activation are shown in Table 1.1. Monoamines do not enter the target cell themselves.

Inactivation and clearance

Catecholamines may be taken up by nerve terminals and reused, or they may be inactivated rapidly by enzymes. There are two main enzymes involved: catechol-

Table 1.1. Effects of stimulation of α- and β-adrenoceptors

α-Adrenoceptors
Vasoconstriction
    Narrowing of arterioles in skin, muscle, kidney and gut, as well as coronary arteries and
        veins
Central nervous system effects
    Alertness, agitation, fear, anxiety; dilatation of pupil
Metabolic effects
    Decreased pancreatic exocrine secretion, increased glycogenolysis
Visceral musculature
    Contraction of stomach, bowel, anal sphincter, trigone; ejaculation
Increased sweating; increased concentration of saliva

β-Adrenoceptors
Vasodilatation
    Affecting coronary, skeletal, pulmonary and renal arteries
Increased heart rate
    Mediated by increased rate, increased contractility, and reduced peripheral resistance
Metabolic effects
    Increased pancreatic exocrine secretion; increased lipolysis and glycogenolysis
Relaxation of bronchial and visceral smooth muscle

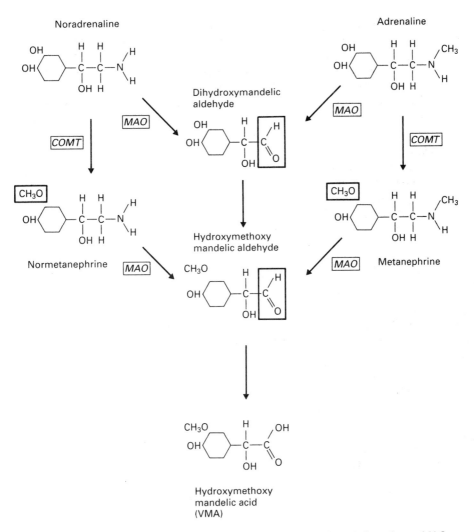

Fig. 1.6. Degradation of catecholamines. COMT, catechol-O-methyltransferase; MAO, monoamine oxidase; VMA, vanillyl mandelic acid.

O-methyl transferase (COMT) and monoamine oxidase (MAO). A small amount is excreted in the urine unchanged. The degradation of catecholamines by these enzymes is summarized in Fig. 1.6.

Derivatives of tryptophan

This group includes 5-hydroxytryptamine (5-HT) and melatonin. 5-hydroxytryptamine is widely distributed throughout the body, whereas melatonin is secreted only by the pineal gland within the brain; 5-HT is also present in the pineal and may or may not be secreted from it. The pineal gland probably has greater physiological importance than is recognized: it has a very rich nerve and blood supply.

Physiology

The concentrations of 5-HT and melatonin in the pineal gland change throughout the day, being responsive to light. It is thought that impingement of light on the retina is transmitted indirectly to the pineal through the adrenergic nervous system. In some seasonal breeders (e.g. birds) the pineal may remain directly sensitive to light, even though it lies within the middle of the brain; 5-HT levels in the pineal are high during daylight. Melatonin is derived from 5-HT and is secreted into the blood stream and into the cerebrospinal fluid (CSF). Melatonin is cleared in the liver.

Biological actions

Relatively little is known, even though it is certain that melatonin is involved in the activation/inactivation of seasonal breeding. This is achieved by melatonin inhibiting gonadotrophin release from the pituitary gland. Melatonin may also be involved in the cyclical or pulsatile release of other hormones — especially those that have a nyctohemeral (night–day) rhythm of secretion, such as GH and prolactin. In addition, there is evidence that the disorientation and drowsiness which accompanies rapid change of time zones (jet lag) can be prevented or treated by the administration of melatonin, suggesting that the hormone has a role in controlling CNS function.

Iodothyronines: thyroxine and triiodothyronine

The secretory cells of the thyroid are gathered into follicles or acini (Fig. 1.7). Their main secretory product is the large protein thyroglobulin (600 000 Da; it constitutes 75% of the protein content of the entire gland). Thyroglobulin is not

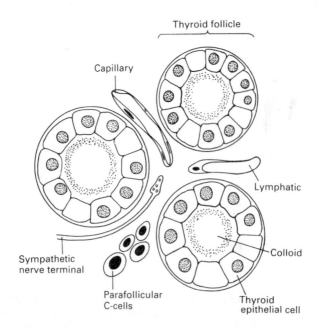

Fig. 1.7. Thyroid histology. The epithelial cells are columnar when the gland is overactive, and flattened when the gland is less active.

normally released into the blood stream, but remains within the colloid of the acinus, acting as a base for the synthesis of the thyroid hormones, thyroxine (T_4) and triiodothyronine (T_3).

Synthesis

The synthesis of T_4 and T_3 involves the incorporation of iodine molecules on to tyrosine molecules, and the fusion of pairs of tyrosine molecules to form iodo-thyronines. The tyrosine needed for this process is cleaved from the parent thyroglobulin molecule, whereas iodide is extracted from the blood and oxidized to iodine by the action of the enzyme thyroid peroxidase. This process is thought to take place at the interface between the acinar cells and the colloid (Fig. 1.8).

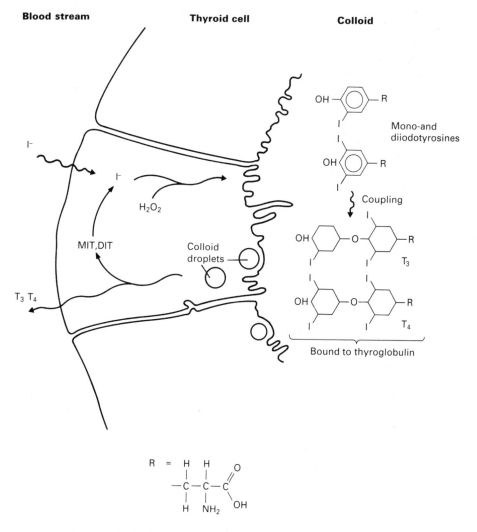

Fig. 1.8. Synthesis of thyroid hormones between the thyroid cell and colloid. T_3, triiodothyronine; T_4, thyroxine. DIT, diiodotyrosine; MIT, monoiodotyrosine.

The conjugation of pairs of iodinated tyrosine molecules and the incorporation of more iodine leads to the formation of T_3 and T_4. These thyroid hormones are then stored in the colloid attached to thyroglobulin. When the gland is stimulated by pituitary TSH, colloid droplets containing T_4 and T_3 enter the thyroid cell, where free T_4 and T_3 are cleaved from thyroglobulin and pass into the circulation. Mono- and diiodotyrosines are secreted in small amounts but do not appear to be biologically active. Only about 20% circulating T_3 is secreted directly by the thyroid. The remainder is derived by the peripheral deiodination of T_4 (Fig. 1.9).

Patterns of release

There is a circadian rhythm of thyroid hormone release, with serum concentrations being very slightly higher in the morning than in the evening. Clearance is slow (half-life being approximately 5 days) and there are no bursts or pulses of secretion.

T_3 and T_4 in the circulation

T_3 and T_4 are thin, planar molecules, and are not water-soluble. They are therefore dependent on attachment to carrier proteins (albumin, prealbumin and thyroid-

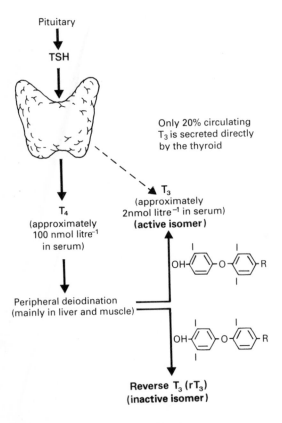

Fig. 1.9. Thyroid hormones in blood.

Table 1.2. The low-T_3 syndrome. Factors associated with increased rT_3 synthesis and with lower T_3 concentrations in blood

Increasing age	Corticosteroid therapy
Female gender	Diabetes mellitus
Obesity	β-Blocker therapy
Ill-health	Liver disease

binding globulin, TBG) for transport in the blood; 99.97% T_4 and 99.5% T_3 are protein-bound in this way. Serum concentrations are higher slightly in winter than in summer.

Interaction with the target cell

It is thought that it is the free, non-protein bound fraction that is biologically active. As the thyroid hormone molecule is small, planar and lipid-soluble, it needs no surface receptor and slips straight into the cell. It passes through the cytoplasm to the nucleus, where it binds directly to DNA to stimulate replication and protein synthesis. Thyroid hormones control cell growth and metabolic activity.

It is thought that T_3 is probably the main active hormone within the target cell, and T_4 may act simply as a prohormone. T_4 which enters target cells is deiodinated (the removal of one iodine atom yields T_3) within the cytoplasm by deiodinases, which are found in most tissues. Some of the T_3 diffuses back into the circulation.

The activity of these deiodinases can be modified: when T_3 is not required by the body, T_4 is deiodinated by an alternative pathway which yields the inactive isomer, reverse T_3 (rT_3). This tends to be formed preferentially, rather than T_3, in a variety of circumstances, and these are listed in Table 1.2. In these circumstances, measured T_3 concentrations in blood tend to be low (the 'low-T_3 syndrome'). Since 80% of circulating T_3 is derived from peripheral iodination, and since this is under the influence of so many factors, it follows that a low T_3 concentration is a poor guide to thyroid status.

Cholesterol derivatives and steroids

There are three main groups of cholesterol-derived steroid hormones:
1 Vitamin D and its metabolites.
2 Adrenocortical hormones.
3 Gonadal hormones.

Vitamin D

Vitamin D is a hormone, not a vitamin. It is synthesized in the skin under the influence of ultraviolet (UV) light and released into the blood stream to act on other tissues. It is only in unusual circumstances, such as inadequate UV light or disease of the gastrointestinal tract, that humans become dependent on vitamin D in the diet. A vitamin is a dietary factor present in trace amounts, but which is essential for normal physiology.

Endogenous vitamin D

The active form of vitamin D is 1,25-dihydroxycholecalciferol (1,25-OHCC). It is also known as calcitriol. 1,25-OHCC is produced from cholecalciferol (called vitamin D_3). Cholecalciferol is synthesized in the skin from cholesterol and 7-dehydrocholesterol, and is then activated in two hydroxylation steps: 25-hydroxylation takes place in the liver, and 1-hydroxylation in the kidney (Fig. 1.10).

Dietary vitamin D

Dietary vitamin D is a complex of closely related sterols, but including 7-dehydrocholesterol. Its main natural source is fish and eggs. It is ingested, and then converted in the skin by the action of UV light into D_3. D_3 is then hydroxylated to 25- and 1,25-OHCC.

Commercial vitamin D

Vitamin D which is available for therapy is called ergocalciferol (vitamin D_2). It is

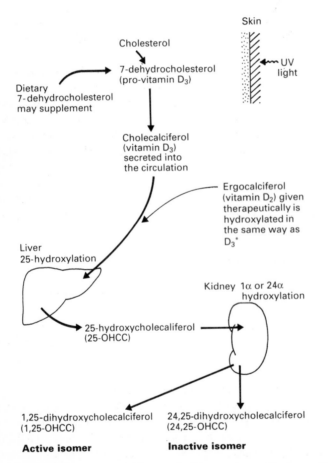

Fig. 1.10. Metabolism of vitamin D. *Note — vitamin D_1 does not exist.

produced from ergosterol (provitamin D_2) using artificial UV light. It is structurally related to cholecalciferol, is hydroxylated in the same way in the body and is equally potent.

1,25-OHCC and 24,25-OHCC

The 1α-hydroxylase which catalyses the synthesis of 1,25-OHCC is stimulated by parathyroid hormone (PTH). It is also stimulated by low serum calcium, and by low serum phosphate. It is inhibited by high calcium and high phosphate. When 1α-hydroxylase is inhibited, 25-OHCC is converted to an inactive isomer — 24,25-OHCC — by 24-hydroxylase in the kidney. The body produces either active 1,25-OHCC or inactive 24,25-OHCC, depending on requirements.

1,25-OHCC in the circulation

As a steroid, this is relatively insoluble in water and is partly protein-bound in blood to vitamin D-binding protein (DBP). DBP has a molecular weight of 53 000 and is secreted by the liver.

Target cell interaction

Steroids resemble thyroid hormones in being planar structures. 1,25-OHCC slips directly into the nuclei of intestinal epithelial cells to stimulate the production of mRNA directly.

The main target organs of 1,25-OHCC are the gut, kidney and bone, but receptors are also found in the pancreas, parathyroid, pituitary and cells of the reticuloendothelial system. Monocytes have receptors for 1,25-OHCC and it is thought that the hormone has a role in controlling the evolution of monocytes and lymphocytes. As osteoclasts (which release calcium from bone) are derived from monocytes and macrophages, it is possible that 1,25-OHCC is responsible for development of osteoclasts.

The details are complex, because there is evidence that macrophages also contain the 1α-hydroxylase necessary to synthesize 1,25-OHCC. The hypercalcaemia of sarcoidosis is caused by increased 1,25-OHCC production by sarcoid granulomata.

Adrenocortical and gonadal steroids

All hormones derived from the adrenal cortex are steroids, but the gonads produce both sex steroids and an increasingly recognized number of peptides. Steroids are synthesized via a complicated cascade, which is illustrated in Fig. 1.11. More details of the different classes of steroids — glucocorticoids (e.g. cortisol), mineralocorticoids (e.g. aldosterone) and sex steroids (e.g. testosterone, oestradiol) — are given in the relevant sections.

Adrenal corticosteroids and gonadal steroids in the circulation

Steroids are relatively insoluble in water and are approximately 95% protein-bound — to albumin and to specific binding proteins such as cortisol-binding globulin (CBG) and sex hormone-binding globulin (SHBG). There is doubt about whether the binding proteins act as mere transport and storage facilities, or whether their role is more specialized. It is possible, especially in the case of sex

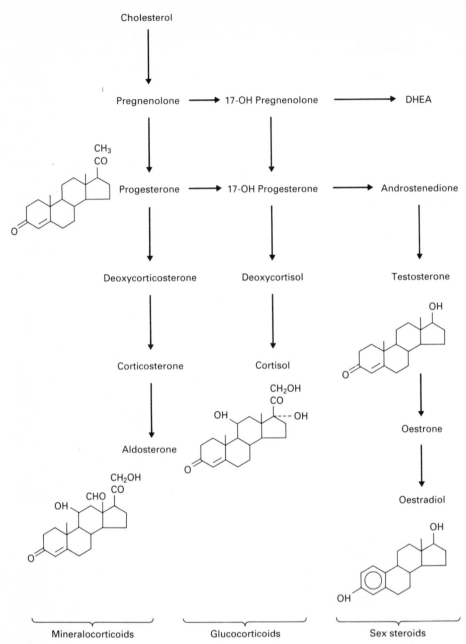

Fig. 1.11. Synthesis of corticosteroids. DHEA, dihydroepiandrosterone.

steroids, that the hormone needs to be protein-bound in order to gain access to the target tissue.

Target cell interaction

One of three things happens after steroids slip into their target cell:

1   They may pass to the nucleus to induce a response.

2   They may be altered to an active metabolite, which then passes to the nucleus to induce a response.

3   They may bind to a cytoplasmic (cytosolic) receptor, and it is the steroid–receptor complex which is transported to the nucleus.

The gonadal steroid testosterone is converted (in some tissues) to a more active metabolite, dihydrotestosterone (DHT).

Inactivation and clearance

Although glucocorticoids may be secreted in a sluggish burst over 20–30 minutes in response to a pulse of ACTH, most changes in blood levels are more slow — over several hours. Inactivation and clearance are not particularly rapid. There is a marked circadian rhythm of adrenal corticosteroids, with high plasma concentrations soon after waking and very low concentrations in the night. Steroids are inactivated in the liver (and also the kidney) by either progressive reduction and oxidation, or by conjugation to glucuronide or sulphate groups. A small amount is excreted in the urine unchanged.

Arachidonic acid derivatives

Derivatives of arachidonic acid are grouped into two main families: the prostaglandin family, including prostacyclin and thromboxane, produced via the key intermediate cyclic endoperoxide, and the leukotriene family (Fig. 1.12). All are closely related structurally, but have a wide variety of different actions. In general their effects are exerted on adjacent cells, or indeed on the cell from which they are derived. They thus usually act as 'paracrine' or 'autocrine' rather than 'endocrine' transmitters. However, prostacyclins certainly act as endocrine agents because they are secreted by one group of cells (the endothelium) and carried in the blood stream to act on other cells elsewhere. For that reason the group is included here.

Arachidonic acid derivatives can be regarded as acting in four main areas: within the central and peripheral nervous systems, on smooth muscle, especially of blood-vessel walls, on the cellular constituents of blood, and finally, in modifying the actions of true endocrine glands.

Synthesis and release

They may be released from the cell or act internally. If released they may act on the cell membrane of the same cell, on adjacent cells, or on distant ones. In the blood stream, these substances are to some extent protein-bound depending on their relative polarity and solubility (prostaglandins F (PGFs) most polar, E (PGEs) intermediate and A (PGAs) least).

Target cell interaction

There are specific cell-surface receptors. Activation triggers a rise in either cAMP or cyclic guanosine monophosphate (cGMP).

Biological actions

They mediate or modify many cellular signals in many tissues. Some of the better known processes are:

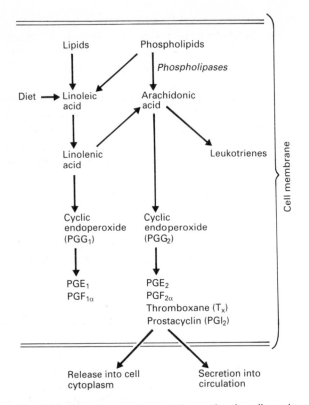

Fig. 1.12. Arachidonic acid metabolism within the cell membrane.

Onset of parturition

Changes in the function of the hypothalamus and pituitary of the fetus at term result in a rise in free cortisol. This triggers the release of $PGF_{2\alpha}$, which acts in concert with oxytocin to induce myometrial contraction. $PGF_{2\alpha}$ can be administered to induce abortion.

Pain sensation

Tissue release of PGE is one of the factors that stimulates the terminals of afferent pain fibres.

Blood-vessel walls, platelets and clotting

Prostacyclins are released from the endothelium, while thromboxanes are derived from arachidonic acid of the platelet cell membrane. They have opposite actions: prostacyclin (PGI_2) inhibits platelet aggregation and causes dilatation of blood vessels, and thromboxanes induce vasoconstriction, platelet aggregation and blood clotting. PGI_2s are tonically released, and as they circulate they prevent platelets aggregating by maintaining elevated cAMP activity within them. However, when vessel walls are damaged, the platelets are stimulated to produce thromboxanes (TXA_2) which release Ca^{++} from calcium stores. This inhibits cAMP production by adenylate cyclase, and the platelets aggregate as a result. There is associated activation of the thrombotic cascade, leading to blood clotting.

Bronchospasm

Many different factors mediate smooth-muscle contraction in the walls of bronchi and bronchioles. Activation of phospholipid metabolism within the mast cell (as a result of immune stimulation) leads to the release of arachidonic acid derivatives. Of these, the leukotrienes cause powerful and sustained contraction of smooth muscle and are the mediators of the late sustained phase of acute asthma.

FACTORS MODIFYING HORMONE ACTION

Control of hormone secretion

In order to induce a specific response at the required time, hormone action has to be regulated. The mechanisms by which it is regulated are many (Fig. 1.13).

Basal secretion

Hormones might be secreted tonically, either continuously (e.g. prolactin) or in a pulsatile manner (e.g. insulin). Lactotrophs and pancreatic β-cells will secrete spontaneously when cultured.

Superadded rhythms

Secretion may be modified by light–dark rhythms, largely as a result of melatonin secretion. There are day–night (nyctohemeral, circadian) rhythms for many hormones, for example ACTH, prolactin, GH and TSH. Circannual rhythms in, for example, TSH are presumably entrained in the same way. The monthly (menstrual) cycles in women of child-bearing age are not apparent in women of non-child-bearing age or in men, and seem to result from a complex servomechanism involving many interrelated factors.

Releasing factors

Hormones may be secreted when required in response to a specific stimulus, which may be nervous (e.g. adrenal medulla) or, more usually, another hormone (releasing factor). Often there are multiple stimuli operating, e.g. the release of insulin in response to parasympathetic nerve stimulation, glucose, and the gut hormone GIP (glucose-dependent insulinotropic peptide).

Stimuli may increase release in one of two ways: (a) the release of hormone stored in secretory vesicles (peptides, catecholamines) — short-burst, rapid effect, and (b) the increased synthesis of hormone — delayed action.

Release-inhibiting factors

Hormones such as prolactin, which are tonically released are under dominant negative control: the prolactin-inhibitory factor is dopamine, secreted by the hypothalamus. Other hormone-secreting cells have release-inhibiting factors, and hormone release is the sum of the effects of positive and negative factors. Thus GH

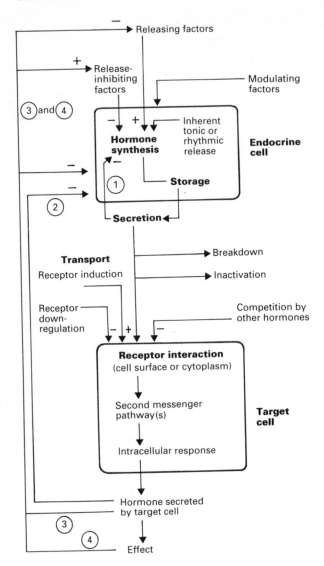

Fig. 1.13. The regulation of hormone action. Negative feedback loops comprise: 1, short-short-loop; 2, short loop; 3, long loop; 4, long-long loop.

is released or not in response to the actions of hypothalamic-releasing (GHRH) and release-inhibiting hormones (GHRIH, somatostatin). Somatostatin also inhibits the release of many other hormones, both in the pituitary (e.g. TSH) and elsewhere (e.g. in the pancreas).

Negative feedback inhibition

Release is inhibited also by negative feedback: the results of hormone secretion act back to inhibit further release.

Short-short loop feedback

The hormone suppresses its own secretion.

Short loop feedback

The hormone suppresses the releasing factor which led to its release.

Long loop feedback

The hormone induces secretion of another hormone by its target tissue, and it is the other hormone that causes feedback inhibition. Examples are common, e.g. feedback of cortisol on corticotrophin-releasing factor (CRF) secretion by the hypothalamus, or testosterone on gonadotrophin-releasing hormone (GnRH).

Long-long loop feedback

The hormone induces a metabolic response which leads to its secretion being suppressed. For example, the secretion of renin by the kidney will be suppressed by retention of sodium and water induced by the (renin-induced) secretion of aldosterone.

Cytokines

Cytokines are members of a large family of peptides. They were originally found in lymphocytes and monocytes, but are now known to be present in many different tissues. They are chemical mediators of inflammatory and immune mechanisms, and act either as paracrines or endocrines.

There are well recognized endocrine consequences of major trauma and disease, and it is likely that many of these are the result of the effect of cytokines. Thus ACTH and cortisol secretion is stimulated by interleukins (IL_1, IL_2 and IL_6) and tumour necrosis factors (TNF), while IL_1 and TNF suppress gonadotrophin secretion and gonadal function. IL_1 and TNF also suppress the pituitary–thyroid axis, as does interferon-γ (INF-γ).

White blood cells also express receptors for many hormones, including ACTH, cortisol, T_3, T_4 and 1,25-OHCC. These connections between the immune and endocrine systems are highly complex and little understood.

Modulation of hormone delivery

It is likely that hormone action is modified by factors altering its delivery to potential target sites. This may be achieved partly by binding proteins, which should not be regarded as simple hormone stores. In some cases hormones such as sex steroids or insulin-like growth factors (IGFs) need to be bound to a specific binding protein to gain access to a target.

Hormone sequestration

The body may induce altered synthesis of binding proteins to result in the temporary inactivation of hormones. Thus, the action of insulin-like growth factor 1 (IGF_1) in the ovary and endometrium is inhibited when the concentration of one of its binding proteins, IGF-BP_1, is increased.

Hormone metabolism

The action of a hormone will be curtailed if its metabolic breakdown is increased.

Receptor induction

Hormones normally act by binding to specific receptors on or in target cells. The number of receptors can be increased by other factors, for example the induction of LH receptors by FSH in the first half of the menstrual cycle — the follicular phase — so that the follicle is capable of responding to the mid-cycle burst of LH secretion.

Receptor down-regulation

When a hormone is secreted in large quantities, it induces down-regulation of its own target organ receptors, thus limiting its action.

Regulation of intracellular response

Little is known of the controls which exist also within the cytoplasm and the nucleus. It is likely that they are just as complex.

SECOND MESSENGERS

When a hormone interacts with a target cell, it may do so by stimulating RNA synthesis directly. This is true of steroids and of thyroid hormones. On the other hand, hormones such as peptides and amines act by binding to a cell surface or a cytosolic receptor to trigger a cascade of cytoplasmic responses. These cytoplasmic responses are mediated by 'second-messenger' systems. There are a number of different second-messenger systems, but it is likely that they all interrelate to give an extra dimension of subtlety to the hormonal message. Hormones which are released in bursts might activate one pathway preferentially; the same hormone acting on the same cell in a tonic fashion may activate a different pathway and induce a different response.

The second messengers can induce cell responses in a number of ways: altered membrane structure and function; activation or inhibition of cytoplasmic rate-limiting enzymes; changes in microtubular protein-movement of intracellular structures; activation or inhibition of RNA transcription or translation. Enzyme activation is achieved largely by inducing the phosphorylation of specific proteins, hence the liberation of phosphate is a key feature of the process.

There are two main intermediary pathways for this intracellular response, and they are interconnected. Both result in liberation of phosphate, and both are intimately involved in changes in intracellular calcium:

1 cAMP (and cGMP) generation.
2 Production of derivatives of phosphatidyl inositol (PI).

Cyclic AMP

Many peptide hormones work through the cAMP system. When the peptide binds to its receptor, it causes the G-protein (which is a membrane-bound part of the adenylate cyclase complex) to trap guanosine triphosphate (GTP). When GTP is bound to the G-protein, it catalyses the formation of cAMP from ATP, thereby

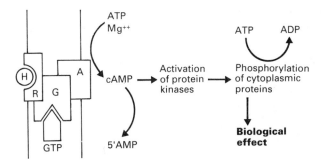

Fig. 1.14. Second messengers: the adenylate cyclase system. A, adenylate cyclase complex; G, G-protein; GTP, guanosine triphosphate; H, hormone; R, receptor.

liberating phosphate. cAMP activates protein kinase and this in turn leads to further enzyme activation by phosphorylation (Fig. 1.14). GTPases form part of the G-protein and these redetach GTP and block the activating process. There are a number of different G-proteins, and this helps confer specificity of response.

Phosphatidyl inositol derivatives

Phosphatidyl inositol is derived from the phospholipid of the cell membrane. It has phosphate groups attached. Receptor activation results in the cleavage of PI into inositol triphosphate (IP_3) and diacylglycerol (DG). IP_3 mobilizes intracellular calcium, which induces a cellular response (see below); DG stimulates protein kinase C to induce enzyme activation by phosphorylation. DG can also be cleaved to liberate arachidonic acid, and hence act as a precursor for the formation of prostaglandins and related substances (Fig. 1.15).

Intracellular calcium

Both the cAMP and the PI system are dependent on intracellular calcium. The concentration of intracellular calcium is one-thousandth that of extracellular fluid. The consequence is that tiny changes in the availability of intracellular calcium are used to trigger intracellular responses to stimulate or suppress enzymes, including enzymes of the cAMP and PI systems. Calcium acts as both an intermediary in these systems and as a factor which controls them. Thus calcium may stimulate or inhibit adenylate cyclase, and it is also integral in the activation of protein kinase C, and in the phosphorylation induced by DG. Calcium will also stimulate the production of arachidonic acid derivatives from phospholipids.

The increase in intracellular calcium may come from increased influx from the extracellular fluid, reduced efflux (calcium is actively pumped from cells continually), or mobilization from intracellular stores, such as calcium bound to the cell membrane, endoplasmic reticulum and the mitochondria.

The calcium may act on enzymes directly or in association with calmodulin, a cytoplasmic protein with a molecular weight of 16 700 Da. Each calmodulin

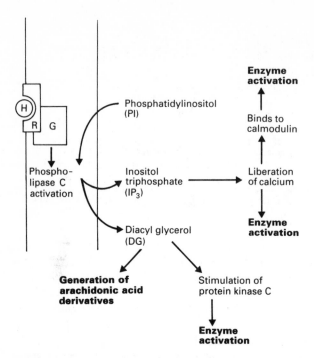

Fig. 1.15. Second messengers: PI derivatives.

molecule can bind four calcium atoms. The calcium–calmodulin complex acts to activate other enzyme systems, including protein kinases.

Specificity resulting from activation of different second messengers

The activation of different receptors by the same hormone may result in a different response by the cell. Thus adrenaline can induce either a stimulatory (via β-receptors) or an inhibitory (via α_2-receptors) response in the same target cell. Binding to β-receptors results in the activation of adenylate cyclase, whereas binding to α-receptors triggers a different cellular response through the use of calcium as a second messenger.

Chapter 2
The Hypothalamus and Pituitary

HYPOTHALAMUS

The hypothalamus lies in the medial, basal part of the forebrain, above the pituitary. It is closely associated with the third ventricle and its cerebrospinal fluid (CSF), and it has extensive vascular and nervous connexions. The main function of the hypothalamus is to act as a homœostatic regulator, much of this being mediated by the release of hypothalamic hormones. There are two types of hypothalamic hormone:

1 *Portal* — Trophic and inhibitory hormones, i.e. those secreted into the hypothalamic–pituitary portal system to stimulate or inhibit the synthesis and secretion of anterior pituitary hormones.

2 *Systemic* — Posterior pituitary hormones, i.e. those transported down elongated axons into the posterior pituitary, to be secreted into the systemic circulation. The hypothalamus is composed of a number of well-defined nuclei. The axons which carry the posterior pituitary hormones are derived from cell bodies in the supraoptic (above the optic chiasm) and paraventricular nuclei (Fig. 2.1).

Hypothalamic hormones

Portal hormones

Hormones released into the hypothalamic–pituitary portal system either stimulate

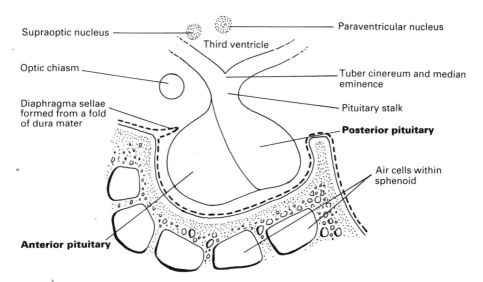

Fig. 2.1. Anatomy of the hypothalamus and pituitary.

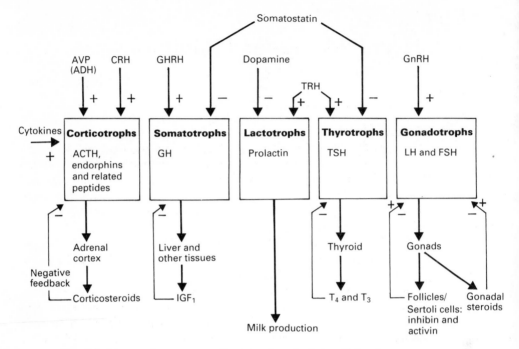

Fig. 2.2. Main mechanisms controlling secretion of anterior pituitary hormones.

hormone synthesis and release by the anterior pituitary (trophic hormones), or inhibit it. The secretion of thyroid-stimulating hormone (TSH), luteinizing hormone (LH) and follicle-stimulating hormone (FSH) by the pituitary is mainly controlled by stimulatory (trophic) hormones: thyrotrophin-releasing hormone (TRH) and gonadotrophin-releasing hormone (GnRH). Prolactin is mainly controlled by an inhibitory hormone (dopamine). Growth hormone (GH) is controlled by both trophic (growth hormone releasing hormone, GHRH) and inhibitory (somatostatin) factors, while the control of adrenocorticotrophic hormone (ACTH) is complex (Fig. 2.2).

Systemic hormones: oxytocin and ADH

The systemic hormones are synthesized in the cell bodies of the supraoptic and paraventricular nuclei, and transported down the axons to the posterior pituitary. The axons have specialized terminals from which the hormones are secreted into the venous sinuses before entering the peripheral circulation. In the axons they are protein-bound to the neurophysins. In fact, both hormones and their neurophysins are derived from a common precursor. The neurophysins are also secreted into the circulation but their physiological function is not known. Oxytocin and antidiuretic hormone (ADH) are both nonapeptides, and are closely related structurally (Fig. 2.3).

Oxytocin

Oxytocin is derived mainly from the paraventricular nucleus. In women it stimulates milk letdown, and may also initiate the myometrial contractions of labour. Its

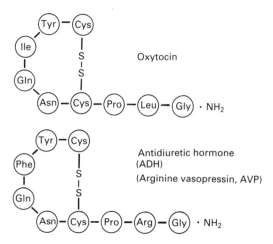

Fig. 2.3. Structure of oxytocin and ADH.

function in men, or in women at other times, is not known. It binds to specific cell-surface receptors on the target organs, and stimulates calcium uptake by the cell. There are no known diseases associated with either excess or deficiency of oxytocin, and women with hypopituitarism who conceive, can go through normal labour.

ADH (arginine vasopressin, AVP)

The main action of ADH is to stimulate water reabsorption in the distal convoluted renal tubule. It interacts with a specific cell-surface receptor to stimulate cyclic adenosine monophosphate (cAMP) release. It stimulates contraction of some smooth muscle (intestine, uterus, coronary arteries), and it elevates blood pressure. It also stimulates hepatic glycogenolysis, and has a role in controlling ACTH release by the anterior pituitary.

ADH is released in response to increasing plasma osmolality (detected by hypothalamic osmoceptors), reduced blood pressure (baroreceptors) and adrenergic stimulation. Nausea is one of the greatest stimuli of ADH secretion, causing plasma levels 5–50 times above normal.

Diseases of the hypothalamus

Structural

Hypothalamic tumours

Craniopharyngioma

Craniopharyngiomas are cysts derived from the remnants of Rathke's pouch. They are not neoplasia but can increase in size progressively as a result of accumulation of the cholesterol-rich fluid they contain. They may present in childhood or adulthood, either as a space-occupying lesion or with evidence of hypothalamic hormone deficiency. Approximately 50% of childhood cranio-pharyngiomas are calcified, and hence apparent on plain skull X-ray. Treatment is by surgical aspiration with, if possible, excision of the cyst capsule. External irradiation is usually given to prevent recurrence. Large craniopharyngiomas found in adults are best left alone, unless they are obviously continuing to expand.

Pituitary tumours

Large pituitary tumours may extend upwards and compress the hypothalamus.

Other tumours

Other tumours may involve the hypothalamus. These include primary intracranial neoplasia (meningioma, glioma, astrocytoma, ependymoma of the third ventricle, pinealloma, teratoma and histiocytosis X), as well as metastases.

Aneurysms and vascular malformations

Large aneurysms and vascular malformations may compress the hypothalamus.

Infiltrations

Hypothalamic function can be impaired by infiltration by a variety of disease processes: tuberculosis, sarcoidosis, syphilis, haemochromatosis, abscesses and fibrosis complicating meningitis.

Functional

Non-structural hypothalamic dysfunction is common but usually temporary. Common examples in women include episodes of oligomenorrhoea, or temporary amenorrhoea after stopping the contraceptive pill. However, more significant dysfunction also occurs — in the absence of any obvious anatomical defect — and may be permanent. Impaired hormone release may be associated rarely with other problems: loss of temperature regulation, hyperphagia or anorexia.

Anorexia nervosa

The weight loss of anorexia nervosa is associated with reduced GnRH secretion and amenorrhoea. When the woman regains her ideal body weight (i.e. body mass index greater than 18), there may be a delay of up to 2 years before her periods return. Serum prolactin concentrations tend to be low in anorexia nervosa, presumably because of increased secretion of the hypothalamic prolactin inhibitory factor, dopamine.

Delayed puberty and small stature

Environmental deprivation and/or ill health can modify hypothalamic function such that growth is slowed and puberty delayed. Stressful events in adulthood can suppress gonadotrophin secretion.

Trauma

Head injury can cause temporary or permanent hypothalamic dysfunction. Reduced secretion of ADH will result in diabetes insipidus, and panhypopituitarism can follow more serious injury.

Idiopathic hypothalamic hormone deficiency

As a result of hypothalamic hormone deficiency, a person may develop deficiency of secretion of one or more pituitary hormones. These may be either true deficiencies, or may represent abnormal control of hypothalamic hormone secretion as much as reduced synthesis. The best-recognized deficiencies are GHRH deficiency — which is the commonest cause of GH deficiency in childhood — and GnRH deficiency as a cause of failure to go through normal puberty. When GnRH deficiency is associated with congenital impairment of the sense of smell (and/or colour blindness) the condition is called Kallman's syndrome. Hypothyroidism may also rarely be the result of idiopathic TRH deficiency, and hypocortisolism can be the result of corticotrophin-releasing hormone (CRH) deficiency, but these are extremely rare. The commonest cause of functional CRH deficiency is hypothalamic and pituitary suppression, caused by prolonged treatment with corticosteroids.

As prolactin secretion by the pituitary is under dominant negative control by hypothalamic dopamine, it is possible that some cases of hyperprolactinaemia are caused by idiopathic dopamine deficiency.

Idiopathic 'hypopituitarism' of the elderly

Loss of hypothalamic function has been described as a degenerative process. The cause is unknown, but it might be ischaemia.

Obesity

There is increasing speculation that abnormal synthesis or release of the peptide, neuropeptide Y (NPY), may be involved in some cases of obesity.

Effects of hypothalamic disease

Structural

Any expanding lesion will result in increasing hypothalamic dysfunction. In addition, occlusion of the foramen of Monro will result in hydrocephalus. Large space-occupying lesions will result in symptoms and signs of raised intracranial pressure.

Hormone deficiency

Portal hormone deficiency

A deficiency of hypothalamic-releasing hormones will result in hypopituitarism. Dopamine deficiency will cause hyperprolactinaemia.

Systemic hormone deficiency: diabetes insipidus

No ill effect seems to accompany oxytocin deficiency. ADH deficiency results in diabetes insipidus (DI). This is a condition in which the body is unable to concentrate urine to conserve water. There are two types of DI: ADH deficiency (cranial DI), and renal tubular insensitivity to circulating ADH (nephrogenic DI). The effects of the two are similar.

Causes

The commonest causes are idiopathic (20%), traumatic (head injury, pituitary surgery), autoimmune (antibodies to hypothalamic nuclei, 10%) and tumours of the hypothalamus. Note that untreated pituitary tumours do not usually cause DI unless they are very big and compress the hypothalamus.

Effect

The inability to concentrate urine will result in progressive dehydration: hyperosmolality of serum with raised blood urea concentration.

Clinical

People with DI complain of thirst and polyuria and will ascribe the polyuria to the thirst, rather than the other way about. They will have nocturia, and will usually be unable to pass the night without having a drink by the bed. Overnight urine volume typically exceeds 1 litre. Idiopathic DI may present at any age, and may be associated with other hypothalamic hormone deficiencies.

In the rare familial DIDMOAD syndrome, affected people have diabetes insipidus (DI), diabetes mellitus (DM), optic atrophy (OA) and deafness (D)

People who have ACTH deficiency as well as DI may not have polydipsia and polyuria until they are given hydrocortisone replacement therapy: hydrocortisone is necessary for proper excretion of a water load.

Diagnosis

DI must be distinguished from other causes of polyuria and dehydration: see Table 2.1. Cranial DI must also be distinguished from nephrogenic DI. Polyuria itself (the passage of large volumes of urine) must be distinguished from frequency (passing urine often). Finally, DI must be distinguished from psychogenic polydipsia (the passage of large volumes of dilute urine because the person has acquired the habit of drinking large volumes of dilute drinks).

Diagnosis depends on demonstrating high plasma osmolality (> 295 mOsmol litre^{-1} in association with low urine osmolality (< 300 mOsmol litre^{-1}). In partial DI urine osmolality may exceed 300 mOsmol litre^{-1}, but will be less than 750 mOsmol litre^{-1}. A person with DI who compensates by drinking enough water

Table 2.1. Causes of polyuria (> 2.5 litres per 24 hours)

Excessive drinking (primary polydipsia)
  Social — beer drinking
  Psychogenic polydipsia
  Hypothalamic disease with abnormal thirst

Absolute or partial ADH deficiency (cranial DI)

Renal tubular insensitivity to ADH (nephrogenic DI)
  Polyuric renal disease; salt-losing nephritis
  Hypercalcaemia, heavy metal poisioning
  Hypokalaemia
  Drug-induced: lithium, demeclocycline
  Inherited

---

may have a normal plasma osmolality, and it is then necessary to demonstrate the effect of water deprivation. The details of the water deprivation test are shown in Table 2.2. It is terminated by giving the synthetic ADH analogue deamino-D-arginine vasopressin (DDAVP), to determine the effect on urine osmolality. DDAVP will cause a rise in urine concentration if the person has cranial DI, but not if the problem is nephrogenic. In cases of doubt it is reasonable to give a trial of treatment with DDAVP.

In some centres ADH assay is possible, and this can be a great help: plasma concentrations will be low in cranial DI and primary polydipsia, and high in nephrogenic DI. The rise in serum ADH which normally accompanies the infusion of hypertonic saline is reduced in cranial DI.

Treatment

DDAVP is given by intranasal spray in doses sufficient to control polyuria. Most people with cranial DI are controlled with between 20 µg each night and 40 µg three times daily. It is very expensive, but there is no alternative.

DDAVP is also used in small doses for nocturnal enuresis in childhood.

Nephrogenic DI might respond to DDAVP if the defect is partial. Tubular sensitivity to ADH can be increased with the sulphonylurea drug chlorpropamide (normally used for diabetes mellitus).

Table 2.2. Water deprivation test

Procedure
No food from midnight, but water allowed. No smoking
Start test at 0800–0900: no food or water allowed
The patient must be closely supervised: extreme thirst can be alleviated by sucking a few ice
    chips
If patient loses > 5% body weight, abandon test
After 6 hours give 2 µg DDAVP intramuscularly or 40 µg intranasally. Allow patient to drink
Takes samples for urine and plasma osmolality at 7 and 8 hours

Each hour:
    Measure urine volume
    Save urine for osmolality measurement
    Take plasma for osmolality measurement
    Weigh patient

Interpretation of results

Peak plasma osmolality (mOsmol litre^{-1})	Peak urine osmolality (mOsmol litre^{-1})	Peak urine osmolality post-DDAVP (mOsmol litre^{-1})	Diagnosis
280–295	> 750	> 750	Normal
> 295	< 300	< 300	Nephrogenic DI
> 295	< 300	> 750	Cranial DI

Equivocal results are often found, especially in people with psychogenic polydipsia who have drunk a lot of water before the test starts.

Hormone excess

Syndrome of inappropriate ADH secretion (SIADH)

The inappropriate secretion of ADH results in retention of excessive water by the renal tubule.

Causes

SIADH has many causes (Table 2.3), and is common. A mild form occurs after general anaesthesia, and is the reason for restricting fluid administration in the first

Table 2.3. Causes of SIADH

Diseases of the chest
Carcinoma of the bronchus
Tuberculosis
Empyema
Chronic obstructive airways disease
Assisted ventilation
Asthma

Intracranial disease
Tumour
Infection
Demyelination
Haemorrhage
Acute psychosis

Drugs increasing ADH secretion
Nicotine
Phenothiazines
Tricyclic antidepressants
Vincristine
Narcotics

Drugs enhancing renal response to ADH
DDAVP
Oxytocin
Indomethacin/non-steroidal anti-inflammatory drugs

Drugs causing SIADH by an uncertain mechanism
Chlorpropamide
Cyclophosphamide
Clofibrate
Carbamazepine

Other tumours
Thymoma
Lymphomas
Leukaemias
Carcinoma of pancreas
Carcinoma of urinary tract

---

24 hours after surgery. SIADH results from resetting of the sensitivity of thoracic baroreceptors and/or hypothalamic nuclei, and it can complicate any disease involving either the chest or the head. In some cases of carcinoma of the bronchus, an ADH-like substance is secreted by the tumour itself.

Effect

Water retention leads to haemodilution, which is asymptomatic when mild but can lead to confusion, convulsions, coma and death.

Diagnosis

There will be biochemical evidence of haemodilution: hyponatraemia, hypo-kalaemia and low plasma urea concentration. The diagnosis can be confirmed by demonstrating low plasma osmolality (< 280 mOsmol litre^{-1}) in the presence of a urine osmolality which is higher.

Hyponatraemia (low serum sodium concentration) occurs commonly in clinical practice. There are two main causes: SIADH and sodium deficiency. Before considering treatment it is essential to assess clinically the person's state of hydration (dehydration implies sodium deficiency, and not SIADH), as well as to collect samples for measurement of serum and urine osmolality, and of urine sodium concentration. Salt depletion is associated with a low urine sodium concentration (unless the problem is caused, as it often is, by the inappropriate use of diuretics). Urine sodium concentration will be normal (20–50 mmol litre^{-1}) in those on diuretics, and in SIADH.

Treatment

Water restriction (to 1000, 800 or 500 ml day^{-1}) will usually cause slow resolution. More rapid correction can be attempted using slow infusion of hypertonic saline, with or without frusemide, in severe cases. If the cause is untreatable (e.g. lung cancer or brain damage), then the condition can be managed by inducing renal tubular damage (iatrogenic nephrogenic DI) by giving a tubular poison, demeclocycline. This should be done only with care.

ANTERIOR PITUITARY

The anterior pituitary develops as an evagination of the roof of the pharynx (Rathke's pouch) which migrates rostrally to join the posterior pituitary growing down from the hypothalamus. It is composed of a compact network of hormone-secreting cells (pituicytes). These cells used to be characterized by histological staining with periodic acid–Schiff–orange G stain into acidophils, basophils and chromophobic cells, but this technique has been replaced by specific immunostaining. There are seven main anterior pituitary hormones recognized (Table 2.4).

ACTH and related peptides are secreted by the same cells (corticotrophs). LH and FSH are secreted by gonadotrophs. The remaining hormones have specific cells of origin: lactotrophs (prolactin), thyrotrophs (TSH) and somatotrophs (GH). These cells are spread more or less evenly through the gland, although lactotrophs (which are the most numerous) tend to be more peripheral.

Table 2.4. Anterior pituitary hormones and their cells of origin

Hormone	Cell of origin
ACTH	Corticotrophs
Endorphins, ACTH-related peptides	Corticotrophs
GH	Somatotrophs
Prolactin	Lactotrophs
TSH	Thyrotrophs
LH	Gonadotrophs
FSH	Gonadotrophs

Blood supply

The blood supply to the pituitary gland is shown in Fig. 2.4. The posterior pituitary is supplied mainly by the paired inferior hypophyseal arteries. The terminals of the neurosecretory axons in the posterior pituitary abut the venous sinuses which carry the hypothalamic hormones into the systemic circulation.

The supply to the anterior pituitary gland is more complicated. The paired superior hypophyseal arteries enter the base of the hypothalamus (median eminence) and form a primary capillary network. Into this network are secreted the hypothalamic trophic and inhibitory hormones which control anterior pituitary function. The capillaries then lead into long, straight venous channels (the hypothalamic–pituitary portal veins) which carry the hypothalamic hormones to the anterior pituitary. The capillaries form into sinuses in and around the pituicytes, and the anterior pituitary hormones are secreted into them. They drain into systemic circulation, mainly via the petrosal veins.

The vessels from the inferior and superior hypophyseal arteries interconnect, and there is retrograde (upwards) flow as well as antegrade (downwards) flow in

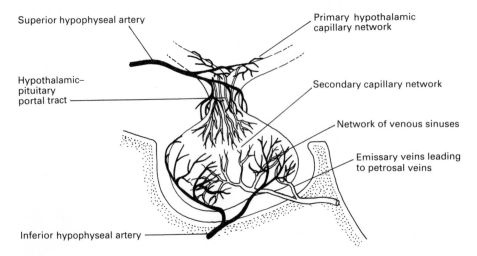

Fig. 2.4. Blood supply of the pituitary.

the pituitary stalk. Blood flows from the pituitary to the hypothalamus, possibly leading to secretion of pituitary hormones into the CSF.

Control of anterior pituitary secretion

The action of the main hypothalamic hormones is summarized in Fig. 2.2. Their action on the pituicytes is modified by other factors:

1 Negative feedback; for example, secretion of TSH will be suppressed by circulating thyroid hormones.

2 Paracrine control. The release of hormones by one pituitary cell may modify the release of hormones by an adjacent one. It is likely that angiotensin II in the pituitary and AVP act in this way.

3 Autocrine control. Hormones released by a secretory cell may act back on the same cell.

4 Other endocrine factors, for example, augmentation of GH secretion by sex steroids, or of prolactin by oestrogens. Cytokines also modulate pituitary function.

Innervation of the pituitary

The posterior pituitary contains nerve axons whose cell bodies lie within the hypothalamus. There are also nerve terminals within the anterior pituitary, but the role of cellular innervation is not known.

Adjacent structures

The top of the pituitary is bounded by a fold of dura, the diaphragma sellae, but in some people it is incomplete. Above this lie CSF, the optic chiasm, the median eminence and the hypothalamus.

To the side of the pituitary lie the cranial nerves III, IV, VI and V (ophthalmic), which run in the medial wall of the cavernous sinus (Fig. 2.5). When a pituitary tumour enlarges sideways rapidly, or behaves in a locally invasive fashion, these

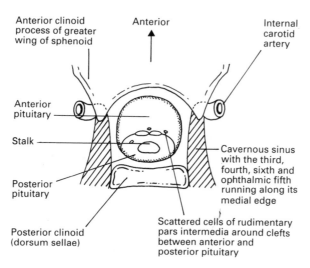

Fig. 2.5. Anatomical relations of the pituitary gland (viewed from above).

nerves may become interrupted. However, the nerves seem to stretch around slow-growing tumours, so that paralysis of the external ocular muscles is uncommon in pituitary disease. The back of the pituitary is bounded by the dorsum sellae, while below it lie the sphenoid air cells.

Hormones of the anterior pituitary

ACTH (adrenocorticotrophin) and ACTH-related peptides

Structure

ACTH is a 39-amino acid straight-chain polypeptide (molecular weight 4500 Da). The N-terminal is essential for receptor binding and biological activity.

Synthesis

It is derived from a large-molecular-weight precursor, pro-opiomelanocortin (POMC) (Fig. 2.6). Pro-opiomelanocortin is broken down in the corticotroph to yield a number of ACTH-related peptides, including β-lipotrophin (β-LPH). β-LPH is without known biological function but it contains within it the structures of the potent morphine-like peptides, β-endorphin and methionine enkephalin (met-enkephalin). The physiological functions of these morphine-like opioid peptides are not known.

ACTH and β-lipotrophin also contain within their length the structures of, respectively, α-MSH (melanocyte-stimulating hormone; ACTH 1–13), β-MSH and corticotrophin-like intermediate lobe peptide (CLIP; ACTH 22–39). α-MSH and β-MSH are secreted in most mammals, but not in humans. The function of CLIP is not known, but it may potentiate insulin secretion by the pancreas.

Control of secretion

ACTH is released by the hypothalamic CRH. Other factors may also be involved

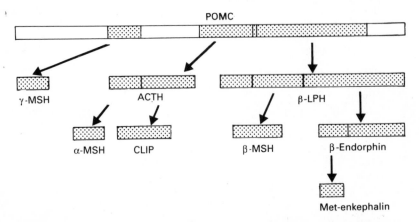

Fig. 2.6. Adrenocorticotrophic hormone (ACTH)-related peptides. CLIP, corticotrophin-like intermediate lobe peptide; MSH, melanocyte-stimulating hormone; POMC, pro-opiomelanocortin. α-MSH and β-MSH do not exist in humans.

(Fig. 2.2), including cytokines. Secretion of ACTH is under three overall influences:

1 Circadian rhythm — high levels in early morning, very low levels in the evening and at night.

2 Stress — physical and psychological stress induces ACTH release.

3 Negative feedback — high plasma glucocorticoid concentrations suppress secretion.

Target cell interaction

ACTH circulates free in plasma, but has a biological half-life of only a few minutes. It interacts with a specific cell-surface receptor in the zona fasciculata and zona reticularis of the adrenal cortex, and stimulates adenylate cyclase.

Biological actions

The main recognized action of ACTH is stimulation of the synthesis and release of cortisol and other corticosteroids from the adrenal cortex.

In humans ACTH is also the main pigmentary hormone. When levels are abnormally high, ACTH causes brownish pigmentation of sun-exposed areas, as well as pressure areas, recent wounds, mucosal membranes, nipples and genitalia.

ACTH is synthesized in tissues other than the pituitary, notably in the neuroendocrine cells of the bronchial mucosa. It is likely to be involved also in modulation of the immune-responsiveness of lymphocytes.

Growth hormone, somatotrophin

Structure

GH is a 191-amino acid polypeptide (molecular weight 21 500 Da) which has considerable structural homology with prolactin, the two being derived from a common ancestral gene.

Synthesis and secretion

GH synthesis and secretion is under dual stimulatory and inhibitory control by hypothalamic GHRH and somatostatin. Many factors stimulate release, but the main ones are sleep, stress and hypoglycaemia. Secretion of GH is augmented by gonadal steroids: increased steroid secretion in early puberty triggers the puberty growth spurt. High GH levels occur in diabetes mellitus, renal failure, anorexia nervosa and starvation.

Target cell interaction and biological action

The main action of GH is to stimulate the formation of insulin-like growth factors (IGFs, formerly called somatomedins) in the liver and, probably, in peripheral tissues as well (Fig. 2.7). IGFs stimulate cell growth. There are two main IGFs: IGF_1 and IGF_2. IGFs circulate in blood bound to large-molecular-weight binding proteins called somatomedin-binding proteins (SBPs). They interact with specific cell-surface receptors to stimulate intracellular tyrosine kinase activity.

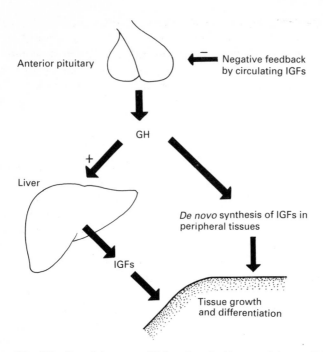

Fig. 2.7. Growth hormone (GH) and insulin-like growth factors (IGFs).

Prolactin

Structure

Prolactin is a 199-amino acid polypeptide (molecular weight 23 000 Da), which is structurally related to GH.

Synthesis and secretion

Prolactin is under tonic negative control by the hypothalamic prolactin-inhibitory factor dopamine. If the pituitary stalk is divided — either through trauma or because it is compressed by a tumour — dopamine cannot obtain access to the lactotrophs and hyperprolactinaemia occurs. There are also one or more hypothalamic prolactin-releasing factors (see Fig. 2.2).

Prolactin is secreted during sleep, and there is also a weak diurnal rhythm, with serum concentrations higher in the morning than later in the day. It is released in response to stress and hypoglycaemia. Oestrogens increase prolactin synthesis and secretion, and levels are very high during pregnancy.

Target cell interaction

Prolactin interacts with specific cell-surface receptors but the second messenger pathway is unknown.

Biological actions

Prolactin is necessary for initiating lactation: a woman whose prolactin is low will not be able to breastfeed. However, prolactin is not needed to maintain lactation and blood concentrations fall to normal within a few weeks in breastfeeding women. It is likely that prolactin has many other physiological roles, but they are unknown. Long-term administration of drugs which lower serum prolactin, such as the dopamine agonist bromocriptine, does not seem to do any harm.

Thyroid-stimulating hormone, thyrotrophin

Structure

TSH, LH and FSH are closely related structurally and, together with the placental hormone human chorionic gonadotrophin (hCG), form the glycoprotein family derived from a common ancestral gene. All four are comprised of two chains, the α- and the β-subunits, which are non-covalently linked (Fig. 1.3). The α-subunit is identical in each, but the β-subunit is specific. TSH has 211 amino acids (28 300 Da).

Synthesis and secretion

Synthesis and secretion are stimulated by hypothalamic thyrotrophin and inhibited by somatostatin. There is a weak circadian rhythm, with TSH concentrations being higher in the middle of the night and lower during the day. There is also a weak annual rhythm, with very slightly higher levels in winter. Apart from these, and apart from the special changes in thyroid function which accompany pregnancy (see p. 74), the serum concentrations of TSH, and of thyroxine are very constant. Secretion of TSH is inhibited by negative feedback by thyroid hormones.

Target cell interaction

TSH binds to a specific cell-surface receptor and stimulates adenylate cyclase.

Biological action

Stimulation of thyroxine and triiodothyronine synthesis and secretion.

Luteinizing hormone and follicle-stimulating hormone

Structure

LH and FSH are structurally related glycoproteins (see above), and are secreted by the same cells; LH (204 amino acids, 28 500 Da) is smaller than FSH (210 amino acids, 34 000 Da).

Synthesis and secretion

Gonadotrophin-releasing hormone (GnRH)
LH and FSH levels are low throughout childhood because release of hypothalamic GnRH is suppressed by some unknown factor. With the onset of puberty there is an increase of GnRH release, and this stimulates synthesis and secretion of both LH and FSH. They are released in bursts, mainly at night, with pulses occurring at approximately 90-minute intervals.

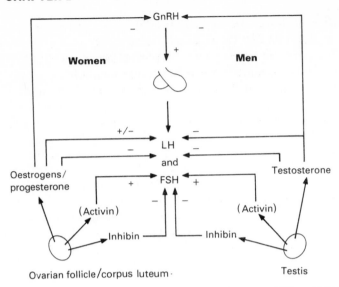

Fig. 2.8. Factors affecting release of luteinizing hormone (LH) and follicle-stimulating hormone (FSH) by the pituitary. GnRH, gonadotrophin-releasing hormone.

Although they are released from the same cells, LH and FSH are not always released together. This is because other factors act to modify the action of GnRH on the gonadotroph. There are at least three such factors: sex steroids, inhibin and activin (Fig. 2.8).

Sex steroids
Oestrogens suppress FSH release in women, but stimulate LH release. Oestrogens and androgens suppress both LH and FSH in men.

Inhibin
Inhibin is a peptide synthesized in the ovarian follicle of women, and the Sertoli cells of the testis. It has an α- and a β-chain (250 amino acids, 32 000 Da), and is structurally related to the cytokine family of transforming growth factor-β (TGF-β). Inhibin causes negative feedback suppression of FSH secretion in both sexes.

Activin
Activin is an isomer of inhibin, and has a completely opposite biological action, stimulating FSH secretion. Activin is widely distributed in many tissues and must have other physiological roles.

Menstrual cycle
The pattern of gonadotrophin secretion in women is fundamentally different because it is cyclical; FSH rises in the follicular phase of the menstrual cycle and stimulates maturation of the follicle which is due to ovulate. The oestrogens secreted by this follicle stimulate a mid-cycle burst of LH secretion, which triggers ovulation.

The climacteric (menopause)

In the male, LH and FSH secretion rise in puberty and remain at the same adult level until senescence. Some men in old age appear to go through a climacteric, analogous to the menopause, but this is exceptional. With the onset of the menopause in women, the ovary becomes unresponsive to LH and FSH; ovulation fails and serum concentrations of LH and FSH rise progressively. Approximately 50% of women suffer hot flushes for several months around the time of the menopause. These irregular bursts of facial flushing coincide with bursts of LH and FSH release, but they are not caused by them: the rise in LH and FSH starts after the beginning of the flush.

Target cell interaction

Like TSH, LH and FSH bind to cell-surface receptors and stimulate adenylate cyclase. The actions of gonadotrophins within the gonad are extremely complex. There is evidence that they are dependent on the synthesis of IGFs.

Biological actions

In the male, LH stimulates the interstitial cell to secrete testosterone. Testosterone and FSH act together on the seminiferous tubule to result in spermatogenesis. In the female, FSH stimulates development of the ovarian follicle, while LH triggers ovulation.

Diseases of the anterior pituitary

The most common problems of the pituitary gland are tumours. Tumours > 10 mm in diameter are called macroadenomas; those < 10 mm are called microadenomas.

Macroadenoma

Tumours of the pituitary may be endocrinologically active (secreting active hormones or hormone fragments) or non-functioning. The commonest hormones secreted are prolactin and GH. ACTH-secreting tumours are third most common. Tumours secreting LH, FSH and TSH are extremely rare. Non-functioning tumours may be associated with hyperprolactinaemia because they can interfere with the access of hypothalamic dopamine to the lactotrophs. Tumours can very occasionally be locally invasive. True malignancy, with metastases, has been reported but is excessively rare.

Microadenoma

Histological microadenomas occur in 30–40% of normal people: only a minute proportion of these behave pathologically by secreting excessive amounts of hormone. Those that do usually secrete prolactin. Prolactin-secreting microadenomas show no general tendency to grow into macroadenomas, and many may regress spontaneously, or after a period of medical treatment.

Other tumours

Because the gland has a generous blood supply, metastases from extracranial tumours often affect the pituitary. The gland can be compressed by meningiomas and other intracranial tumours.

Infiltrations

The gland may be affected by any of the infiltrations which affect the hypothalamus.

Vascular disease

The pituitary gland can be compressed by an aneurysm of the internal carotid artery.

Sheehan's syndrome

Sheehan's syndrome is the name given to post-partum infarction of the pituitary gland. This occurs if a woman has a torrential post-partum haemorrhage (sufficient to cause hypotension and to be life-threatening). In such circumstances the pituitary gland, which is enlarged and very vascular at the time of delivery, is susceptible to total infarction. The woman will not lactate and later develops secondary and permanent amenorrhoea, with the loss of all body hair. If undiagnosed and untreated, she may die from cortisol or thyroxine deficiency. The condition is very rare in countries in which specialist expertise (including blood transfusion) is generally available for the management of complicated labour. The prolactin concentration in Sheehan's syndrome is low, unlike that in all other pituitary disease.

Pituitary apoplexy

Pituitary tumours may infarct when they outgrow their blood supply. This is called pituitary apoplexy, and usually presents with sudden severe headache or collapse. It can mimic subarachnoid haemorrhage and is regarded as a neurosurgical emergency.

Effects of pituitary tumours

Structural

Upwards extension

Optic chiasm

The nerves which cross the midline in the optic chiasm come from the medial part of each retina. The visual field defect caused by compression of the optic chiasm is bitemporal hemianopia, with macular sparing (Fig. 2.9). If compression affects only the lower fibres in the chiasm, the defect produced is an upper quadrantopia because the lower fibres in the chiasm come from the lower part of the retinae. The fibres from cones in the retina are more susceptible to external pressure than those from rods, and so colour vision (especially red vision) is lost before black and white vision.

Further upwards extension may affect the hypothalamus, causing DI and other hypothalamic defects. If the third ventricle is involved, the tumour can cause

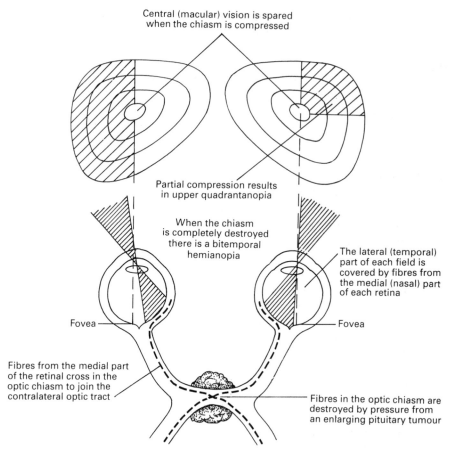

Fig. 2.9. Damage to the optic chiasm by a pituitary tumour causes bitemporal hemianopia.

raised intracranial pressure and hydrocephalus. Very large tumours can occupy large areas of the brain.

Sideways extension

If a tumour expands rapidly (e.g. from haemorrhage) it may cause external ophthalmoplegia by compressing the third, fourth or sixth cranial nerves. This does not tend to happen with slow-growing tumours unless they are locally invasive; instead, the nerves stretch around the tumour.

Downwards extension

Tumours growing downwards are often asymptomatic. However, they can erode into the nasopharynx and present as a 'nasal polyp'. Such tumours can be complicated by devastating bacterial meningitis.

Table 2.5. Clinical signs of cortisol deficiency

General ill-health
Malaise, lassitude
Nausea, vomiting
Abdominal pain
Weight loss, weakness
Dizziness from volume depletion
Reduced resistance to intercurrent illness
Signs of hypoglycaemia

Headache

Some tumours cause persistent severe headache and some are pain free. The headache is thought to derive from nerve terminals in the surrounding dura mater, but does not seem to relate to tumour size. Headache may persist after otherwise effective surgery.

Hormone deficiency

As a pituitary tumour expands it compresses surrounding normal tissue and causes varying degrees of hormone deficiency (hypopituitarism). It is traditionally said that LH, FSH and GH secretion are the earliest to be affected, but exceptions to the rule are so common that this is best forgotten. ADH deficiency (DI) does not occur in untreated pituitary tumours unless they involve the pituitary stalk, or unless they are very big and involve the hypothalamus. DI is usually a feature of disease of the hypothalamus, and not the pituitary.

LH, FSH and GH deficiency are not life-threatening and can be investigated at leisure. However, deficiency of ACTH and TSH are potentially serious and need to be established or excluded as a relative emergency.

ACTH deficiency

Clinical

ACTH deficiency causes reduced glucocorticoid (cortisol) secretion by the adrenals. Mineralocorticoid secretion (aldosterone) is preserved because it is

Table 2.6. Biochemical features of ACTH/cortisol deficiency

Simple measurements: potentially available in an emergency
Hyponatraemia (with natriuria)
High blood urea (haemoconcentration)
Hyperkalaemia
Hypercalcaemia
Eosinophilia

Results not available as an emergency
Serum cortisol concentration
Cortisol response to Synacthen (see Fig. 2.10)
Cortisol response to hypoglycaemia (see Fig. 2.10)

ACTH assay is difficult and expensive and is not necessary for clinical purposes under dominant control by the renin–angiotensin system. The effects of cortisol deficiency are listed in Table 2.5. When severe, ACTH deficiency will result in collapse, coma and death.

Diagnosis

The biochemical features of cortisol deficiency are listed in Table 2.6. In an emergency, blood should be taken and stored for later assay of cortisol. A result of < 250 nmol litre^{-1} in someone who is acutely ill indicates cortisol deficiency. Results between 250 and 600 nmol litre^{-1} are equivocal. In response to stimulation with tetracosactrin (Synacthen) or hypoglycaemia, the plasma cortisol normally rises to > 600 nmol litre^{-1} (Fig. 2.10).

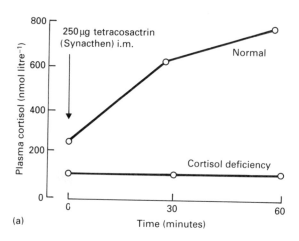

(a)

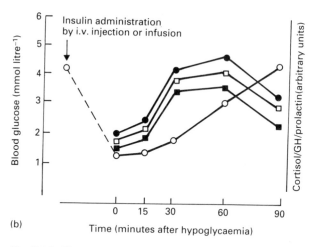

(b)

Fig. 2.10. The short Synacthen and hypoglycaemia stress tests. (a) Short Synacthen test. (b) Hypoglycaemia stress test. Normal response of serum cortisol (●——●), growth hormone (GH) (□——□) and prolactin (■——■) to hypoglycaemia [blood glucose (○——○) < 2.2 mmol litre^{-1}] induced by insulin.

Table 2.7. Emergency management of ACTH/cortisol deficiency

Bed rest

Encourage oral fluids and carbohydrate, if the patient is able to tolerate them

Intravenous infusion of normal saline: 1 litre in 1st hour, 0.5 litres in 2nd, 3rd and 4th hours, more slowly thereafter. The infusion rate needs to be reduced appropriately in children and in those liable to congestive cardiac failure. Saline infusion is just as important in the initial management as hydrocortisone.

Parenteral (i.v. or i.m.) hydrocortisone 50–100 mg 6-hourly until infusion is discontinued. Continue with oral doses of hydrocortisone, reducing to 20 mg three times daily, and then to the maintenance dose.

Note: Hydrocortisone is simply another name for cortisol

Treatment

Acute ACTH or cortisol deficiency is managed as outlined in Table 2.7. Maintenance therapy involves twice-daily oral hydrocortisone, usually in doses between 10 mg b.d. and 20 mg b.d. Mineralocorticoid replacement therapy with fludrocortisone (0.05–1.0 mg on alternate days or daily) is not necessary when cortisol deficiency is the result of pituitary disease because aldosterone secretion by the adrenal is maintained.

TSH deficiency

Clinical

The person will be clinically hypothyroid.

Diagnosis

The serum thyroxine (T_4) concentration will be at or below the lower limit of the reference range (less than approximately 60 nmol litre^{-1}). TSH measurement is of no extra benefit: it may be either frankly low or in the normal range. The TRH test (Fig. 2.11) has been used widely to document TSH reserve but is now redundant. Similarly, triiodothyronine (T_3) assay is of no value because there are many reasons for low serum T_3 concentrations, apart from hypothyroidism (see p. 13).

Treatment

Treatment involves giving oral T_4 in doses between 50 and 150 µg daily (occasionally more). Liothyronine (T_3) can be given parenterally if the person is unable to take tablets because of the severity of their illness.

GH deficiency

Clinical

A child who is deficient in GH will grow slowly. An adult may have no obvious clinical deficit, but GH deficiency leads to protein wasting, with thinner skin and muscle weakness, and the osteoporosis which is a feature of untreated hypopituitarism.

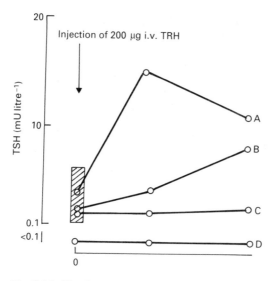

Fig. 2.11. The thyrotrophin-releasing hormone (TRH) test. Normal range for serum TSH is 0.8–4.7 mU litre^{-1}. A, normal; B, partial deficiency (pituitary or hypothalamic disease); C, TSH deficiency; D, TSH suppression, as in Graves' disease. In Graves' disease, serum TSH is undetectable (< 0.1 mU litre^{-1}). The TRH test was evolved before TSH assays were sensitive enough to detect levels below 1.0 mU litre^{-1}. It is now largely obsolete.

Diagnosis

The assessment of small stature in childhood is discussed in detail elsewhere (see pp. 182–5). It can be very difficult. GH deficiency can only be excluded reliably by demonstrating:

1 Normal growth velocity.

2 GH concentration of > 20 mU litre^{-1} basally, during sleep or in response to hypoglycaemia (see hypoglycaemia stress test, Fig. 2.10).

As GH mainly acts by stimulating IGF$_1$ synthesis, IGF$_1$ assay has also been advocated, but it is not widely used.

Treatment

GH deficiency in childhood is treated by two or three weekly subcutaneous or intramuscular injections of biosynthetic hGH (0.5 U kg^{-1} week^{-1}). Before 1986, children were treated with GH extracted from postmortem pituitaries. This practice was discontinued when very occasional (six out of 1908 children treated with GH in the UK and Eire between 1959 and 1985) cases of Creutzfeld–Jakob disease led to the suggestion that the extracted material might have been contaminated by pathogenic slow viruses.

LH and FSH deficiency

LH and FSH are both under the control of the hypothalamic releasing hormone GnRH. Deficiency of one is usually accompanied by deficiency of the other. A man who is producing spermatozoa and a woman who is ovulating may be assumed to have normal reserves of LH and FSH.

Clinical (male)

A boy with gonadotrophin deficiency will fail to go into puberty, but will continue to grow linearly (unless there is associated GH deficiency). He will become tall and eunuchoid (long arms and legs, Figs 2.12, 2.13) but remain hypogonadal.

A man who is LH-deficient will have a low testosterone, resulting in reduced libido and reduced volume of ejaculate, partly from decreased spermatogenesis and partly from decreased secretion by the prostate and seminal vesicles. FSH deficiency also results in reduced spermatogenesis, with small, soft testes. Testis size is assessed using a Prader orchidometer — a series of ovoids of different volumes. The normal adult testis is 15–25 ml or more in volume. Testosterone deficiency may lead to loss of body muscle mass and of beard hair. Loss of axillary and pubic hair will occur if the man is also ACTH-deficient and hence has no adrenal androgens either.

Clinical (female)

A child with LH and FSH deficiency will fail to go into puberty. A premenopausal woman will fail to ovulate and will develop secondary amenorrhoea. A postmenopausal woman will have no ill-effects.

Diagnosis

Deficiency in the male is confirmed by demonstrating normal or low concentrations of serum LH in association with low serum testosterone or azoospermia. There is no simple way of confirming LH and FSH deficiency in the premenopausal female, but low serum concentrations in a woman with amenorrhoea and other evidence of pituitary disease is fairly conclusive. Provocative testing with the hypothalamic hormone GnRH (luteinizing hormone-releasing hormone, LHRH), similar to the TRH test (Fig. 2.11) has no clinical value (but see p. 192). Gonadotrophin deficiency is more easily demonstrated in elderly women because the serum LH and FSH will be low, when they should be high.

Treatment

Child

The boy who is gonadotrophin-deficient will need injections of testosterone to induce secondary sexual characteristics. Girls require treatment with cyclical oestrogens (e.g. with an oral contraceptive preparation) to induce breast development and regular uterine bleeding.

Man who is not particularly interested in fertility

He will require lifelong treatment with testosterone, both to maintain normal sexual activity, and to prevent osteoporosis. Oral preparations (such as capsules of testosterone undecanoate) are only partially effective. Monthly injections with mixed esters (Sustanon or Primoteston) are effective but can be painful and

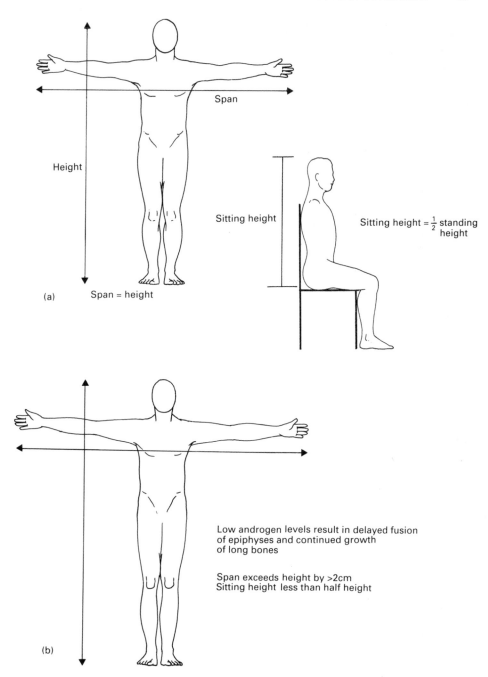

Span

Height

Sitting height

Sitting height $= \frac{1}{2}$ standing height

(a)   Span = height

Low androgen levels result in delayed fusion of epiphyses and continued growth of long bones

Span exceeds height by >2cm
Sitting height less than half height

(b)

Fig. 2.12. (a) Normal and (b) eunuchoidal stature.

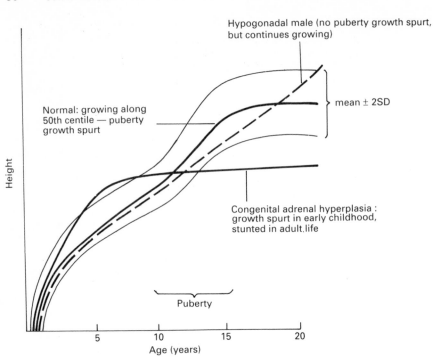

Fig. 2.13. Height chart demonstrating normal and hypogonadal growth, as well as congenital adrenal hyperplasia.

inconvenient. Six-monthly implants of testosterone (200–600 mg) are preferred by some. Implantation of testicular prostheses for cosmetic reasons may also be necessary.

Man who wants children
He requires treatment for 6 months with twice-weekly injections of hCG (which is LH-like) and thrice-weekly injections of MG (human menopausal gonadotrophin: extracted from the urine of menopausal women — FSH-like) (Fig. 2.14). The dose and frequency of injections are empirical and have not been subjected to scientific study. The treatment is effective but expensive, inconvenient and painful. Extra specimens of semen produced at the end of this treatment should be frozen and stored for use in artificial insemination (AI) for those couples who might want further children.

Woman who does not want children
Depending on her age, wishes and social circumstances, a woman will require oestrogen replacement therapy for two reasons: to preserve libido and normal secondary sexual characteristics, and to prevent osteoporosis.

Woman who wants children
To induce ovulation, she will require cyclical injection treatment with FSH and

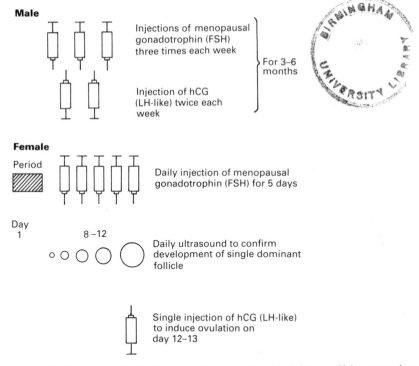

Fig. 2.14. Treatment of infertility caused by gonadotrophin deficiency. If the woman has amenorrhoea, treatment can be started at any time.

LH-like preparations. FSH (i.e. hMG) is given by injection on days 7–12 of the menstrual cycle. Follicle development is monitored by ultrasound. If there is a single dominant follicle, it is induced to ovulate by the mid-cycle administration of hCG (LH-like) (Fig. 2.14). If follicle development is not carefully monitored there is a risk of inducing multiple ovulation, with multiple (non-identical) pregnancies.

Prolactin deficiency

Low serum prolactin concentrations (< 80 mU litre^{-1}) occur in only three circumstances:

1 Pituitary infarction (Sheehan's syndrome).
2 Starvation (including anorexia nervosa).
3 Treatment with drugs that lower prolactin.

Hormone excess

ACTH — Cushing's disease

Harvey Cushing was an American neurologist who described the features of this condition in 1932. There are four main causes (see p. 96), but excess pituitary ACTH secretion is the commonest. Pituitary Cushing's is called Cushing's disease, whereas other forms are called Cushing's syndrome.

Excess ACTH causes bilateral adrenal hyperplasia, and the hyperplastic glands secrete glucocorticoids (mainly cortisol), mineralocorticoids (deoxycorticosterone — but not aldosterone, which is controlled by the renin–angiotensin system and not by ACTH) and sex steroids (mainly androgens).

Clinical

Most of the features of the condition are the result of excessive corticosteroid secretion (see Table 4.2 and Fig. 4.7). In pituitary-dependent Cushing's disease, the increased ACTH may also cause pigmentation of the skin and mucous membranes. The pituitary adenoma may also cause local effects, but this is uncommon because ACTH-secreting pituitary tumours are usually small.

Diagnosis

The diagnosis is both clinical and biochemical. Clinical features are given in Table 4.2 and Fig. 4.7.

Biochemical tests depend on demonstrating increased cortisol excretion (24-hour urine) and abnormal responses in dynamic tests. These dynamic tests are based on demonstrating loss of the normal controls of ACTH secretion (loss of feedback suppression by dexamethasone; loss of stimulation by hypoglycaemia). Cortisol is assayed instead of ACTH because it is easier and cheaper. Biochemical diagnosis falls into three stages:

1 Simple outpatient tests to exclude Cushing's syndrome:
(a) 24-hour urine cortisol excretion (should be < 330 nmol day^{-1}).
(b) Overnight dexamethasone suppression test: 1 mg oral dexamethasone at midnight normally suppresses 9 a.m. serum cortisol to < 60 nmol litre^{-1}.
2 Definitive tests to prove Cushing's syndrome:
(a) 48-hour (low-dose) dexamethasone suppression test: 0.5 mg dexamethasone orally each 6 hours for 48 hours.
Urine cortisol on 2nd day should be < 60 nmol per 24 hours.
Plasma cortisol at 48 hours should be < 60 nmol litre^{-1}.
(b) Hypoglycaemia stress test (insulin tolerance test):
No rise in plasma cortisol after hypoglycaemia
(blood glucose < 2.2 mmol litre^{-1}).
3 Diagnosis of cause — a pituitary cause is suggested by:
(a) Pituitary tumour on skull X-ray.
(b) Plasma ACTH which is at the upper end of the reference range (80 ng litre^{-1}) or slightly high.
(c) Partial suppression of plasma cortisol in high-dose dexamethasone suppression test (2.0 mg orally for 48 hours).
(d) Exaggerated response of cortisol to intravenous CRH.

Treatment

Drugs to reduce ACTH secretion
Very occasionally drugs such as bromocriptine and cyproheptadine have been shown to control pituitary Cushing's by reducing ACTH secretion.

Drugs to reduce cortisol secretion by the adrenal
There are three drugs available: metyrapone, aminoglutethimide and opDDD (mitotane).

Ablative treatment of the pituitary
The pituitary tumour can be treated by transsphenoidal or transfrontal surgery, or by internal or external irradiation. Transsphenoidal excision of the pituitary tumour is the treatment of choice and results in cure in 60–80% of cases.

Adrenalectomy
If it is not possible to eliminate excessive ACTH secretion completely, the effects of increased corticosteroid secretion can be reversed by removing both adrenal glands. The person will be dependent thereafter on replacement therapy, but should otherwise be well.

Nelson's syndrome
After bilateral adrenalectomy there is a risk of the pituitary adenoma suddenly increasing in size. The resultant tumour can become aggressive and locally invasive; ACTH levels rise very high, causing deep skin pigmentation. The risk of this happening has been estimated as 20–30%, but it is unlikely to occur if the person has had previous pituitary surgery. The condition is known as Nelson's syndrome. It may, or may not, be preventable by pituitary irradiation.

Comment
Cushing's disease can be a very difficult condition to diagnose, and frustrating to manage. As it is also extremely rare (fewer than five cases per million population per year), it should be managed only in specialist units.

GH — acromegaly/gigantism
If a pituitary tumour secretes GH in a child, or in someone whose epiphyses have not fused because of hypogonadism in adolescence, it will cause a generalized increase in body size and stature — gigantism. If the tumour occurs in an adult, it causes acromegaly. In acromegaly excessive growth is confined to the soft tissues (skin, subcutaneous tissue and viscera) and to certain bones (especially hands, feet and jaw).

Clinical
The facial appearances are characteristic, with a large jaw, nose and supraorbital ridge, and thickening of the subcutaneous tissues causing prominent nasolabial folds and furrows. The hands are square and spade-like, while the feet are wide and podgy. The disease is usually very slow in evolution, but the person may recall having to have rings enlarged, and bigger shoe (or hat) sizes. Increased greasy sweating is a characteristic feature.

The increased body size and altered bone structure cause a predisposition to osteoarthritis. About one-third have hypertension and one-tenth have hypercalcaemia (from associated hyperparathyroidism). The hypertension can be associated with ischaemic heart disease, but acromegalics are also susceptible to a specific acromegalic cardiomyopathy. They may also have diabetes, because GH acts as an insulin antagonist.

GH-secreting pituitary tumours are sometimes small, but can be very large. They may cause hypopituitarism and other pressure effects. Some GH-secreting tumours also secrete prolactin. The symptoms and signs of hyperprolactinaemia are described below.

Giants have features of acromegaly in association with overall increased stature. As they can only develop gigantism if they are hypogonadal, they will be eunuchoid in proportion (see Fig. 2.12), with relatively long arms and legs and a span which is greater than height.

Diagnosis

The diagnosis is clinical and biochemical. Biochemical diagnosis depends on demonstrating elevation of serum GH concentration. As GH is normally secreted in bursts, there is no true upper limit of normal, but concentrations consistently 10 mU litre^{-1} would be diagnostic in someone with clear signs. The diagnosis can be confirmed with a glucose tolerance test: GH is normally suppressed to < 1 mU litre^{-1} after 75 g oral glucose. In acromegaly the GH may be only partly suppressed, may be unaffected or may even rise (Fig. 2.15).

Slightly high GH concentrations and reduced response to glucose can be found also in chronic renal failure, thyrotoxicosis, diabetes mellitus, anorexia nervosa and starvation.

Measurement of serum IGF$_1$ concentration is being used increasingly as a marker of increased GH secretion.

Treatment

1   Drugs to reduce GH secretion:

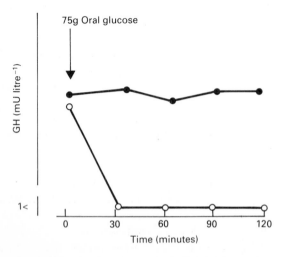

Fig. 2.15. Diagnosis of acromegaly. Normal (○——○); acromegaly (●——●).

(a) Bromocriptine — a dopamine-receptor agonist which causes some reduction in GH secretion and also in tumour size in some but the benefit, when it occurs, is only partial.

(b) Somatostatin — a synthetic GH release-inhibiting hormone which will lower GH (and IGF_1) concentrations to some extent in over 50% of patients. It is expensive and has to be given by multiple daily injections or by continuous subcutaneous infusion.

2 Ablative treatment of the pituitary tumour — the tumour can be treated by transsphenoidal or transfrontal surgery, or by internal or external irradiation. The larger the tumour, the harder it is to cure.

Comment

It is reasonable to suspect that Goliath was suffering from pituitary disease. Such a giant would have been big, but not very strong. He could have had hypogonadism, cortisol deficiency with postural hypotension, myopathy, hypercalcaemia, diabetes mellitus and bitemporal hemianopia!

Prolactin

Prolactinomas are the most common sort of pituitary tumour. Large tumours (> 1 cm diameter) are called macroprolactinomas. They behave in a fundamentally different way from microprolactinomas (< 1 cm), and have a different significance and prognosis.

Macroprolactinoma

Large prolactin-secreting tumours affect men and women equally, and may present either with the effects of hyperprolactinaemia or with the effects of the pituitary tumour itself.

Microprolactinoma

Small prolactin-secreting tumours are extremely common. Sequential post-mortem studies have revealed that they may be present in over 10% of the population, even though they are clinically apparent only in a tiny minority. They present much more commonly in women than in men — usually because of the galactorrhoea and menstrual disturbance they cause. Their cause is unknown but some seem to be self-limiting, suggesting that they may arise from a functional abnormality such as defective release of hypothalamic dopamine.

It is important to recognize that microprolactinomas are not just early macroprolactinomas. They do not tend to grow, even when left untreated.

Clinical

Prolactinomas cause hyperprolactinaemia. Hyperprolactinaemia is associated with a number of typical symptoms and signs (Table 2.8). Note that prolactin does *not* cause gynaecomastia — it causes galactorrhoea (inappropriate milk production). Furthermore, prolactin will only cause galactorrhoea if the breast has been primed with oestrogens: it is uncommon in post-menopausal women, women with long-standing amenorrhoea, and men.

Table 2.8. Symptoms and signs of hyperprolactinaemia

Defective gonadotrophin release and hypogonadism
Women
    Oligo- or amenorrhoea
    Infertility
    Loss of libido
    Dyspareunia from hypo-oestrogenism

Men
    Reduced volume of ejaculate
    Oligo- or azoospermia
    Loss of libido
    Impotence

Effect of prolactin on oestrogen-primed breast
Galactorrhoea — which may be heavy enough to wet clothes, or may be so slight that it is
    only found on examination

Non-specific symptoms
Malaise
Difficulty losing weight
Feeling of bloatedness

The main effects of prolactin result from the hypogonadism it induces. If hypogonadism remains untreated for many years, there is a risk of osteoporosis and fractures in later life.

Other causes of hyperprolactinaemia

Hyperprolactinaemia occurs in a number of other conditions: pregnancy, hypothyroidism, drugs (phenothiazines, metoclopramide, domperidone, methyldopa, haloperidol, opiates) and chronic renal failure, as well as acutely — in response to physical stress and hypoglycaemia.

Diagnosis

Diagnosis depends on demonstrating that basal serum prolactin concentrations are consistently elevated. Unfortunately, there is no clear cut-off between normal and abnormal and experts disagree about what constitutes 'hyperprolactinaemia'. Most would accept that concentrations are high when they are consistently over 700 mU litre^{-1} in women and 500 mU litre^{-1} in men. Special tests of prolactin secretion are unhelpful.

Treatment

The cells of prolactin-secreting tumours nearly always retain their sensitivity to suppression by dopamine and dopamine-receptor stimulating drugs. The dopamine agonist bromocriptine has been widely used for this purpose for almost 20 years. In doses of 2.5 mg b.d. to 10 mg t.d.s., it suppresses prolactin secretion and usually cures symptoms. In addition, treatment with bromocriptine and other dopamine-receptor agonists will cause most prolactinomas to shrink — even very large ones. It is the treatment of choice and should always be tried in preference to surgery. None the less, a minority of prolactinomas will prove resistant to drug therapy and surgery may be necessary.

Normoprolactinaemic galactorrhoea

It is quite common for women to notice galactorrhoea but for there to be nothing endocrinologically wrong — especially if they have regular periods. It is important to make sure that such cases are handled sensibly from the start: it is very easy for them to be frightened unnecessarily by discussion of the possibility of pituitary tumours, and many have unnecessary investigations.

A woman with galactorrhoea but with regular periods should have her serum prolactin measured twice, and she should have a plain lateral skull X-ray. If these tests are normal, she should be reassured and discharged. If she has amenorrhoea or oligomenorrhoea, she should have a computed tomography (CT) scan of the pituitary gland. If she has hyperprolactinaemia, or has a pituitary adenoma, she needs to be fully evaluated in a specialist endocrinology centre.

Assessment of pituitary tumours

Summary

Pituitary tumours cause three sorts of problem:
1 Space-occupying lesion compressing adjacent structures.
2 Hypopituitarism from compression of surrounding normal gland.
3 Excessive hormone secretion — usually ACTH, GH or prolactin.

If a tumour is suspected, two things must be done urgently. The first is to determine how big it is, and whether it is compressing the optic chiasm. The second is the exclusion of ACTH and TSH deficiency. Deficiency of other hormones is less critical. The biochemical tests used in full assessment are listed in Table 2.9.

Treatment of pituitary tumours

Urgency of treatment

If a tumour is causing compression of the chiasm or other significant local pressure effect, it must be treated urgently. If it is causing deficiency of ACTH or TSH, replacment therapy with hydrocortisone and thyroxine should be commenced while other investigations are completed. Tumours which are not growing in size, and which are causing no clinically significant pressure or endocrine effects, may be left untreated and simply observed. Many young women with a microprolactinoma can be left untreated if these conditions are fulfilled.

Trial of medical therapy

In cases of prolactinoma, a trial of therapy with bromocriptine, or other dopamine receptor agonist, should be tried first. This is true even of very big tumours. Bromocriptine may also be tried in GH-secreting tumours, but the response is not so good. An alternative therapy for GH-secreting tumours is the use of somatostatin. It requires multiple injections but is effective in over 50% of cases. Medical therapy of ACTH-secreting tumours rarely works.

Table 2.9. Biochemical assessment of hypopituitarism

Hormone	Basal tests	Dynamic tests
ACTH	Hyponatraemia Hyperkalaemia Cortisol < 250 nmol litre^{-1}	Synacthen test Insulin stress test (IST)
TSH	T$_4$ low TSH low or inappropriately in normal range	TRH test (of little value)
GH	Deficiency excluded if random or sleep GH > 20 mU litre^{-1}	Hypoglycaemia stress test (insulin tolerance test)
LH/FSH (male)	Testosterone low LH low or inappropriately in normal range Azoospermia with low FSH	GnRH (LHRH) test (of little value)
LH/FSH (female)	Anovulation and amenorrhoea in someone with other evidence of pituitary disease	

The injection of synthetic hypothalamic releasing hormones, TRH and LHRH (GnRH), has been widely used to demonstrate reduced reserve of the pituitary hormones TSH, LH and FSH, but partial responses are difficult to interpret. GRH and CRH tests have also been used to assess the response of GH and ACTH, but are not routine.
* Assessment of ACTH reserve on basal blood samples is very difficult, but serum cortisol should be greater than 250 nmol litre^{-1} at 0900 hours in someone who is acutely ill.

Transfrontal surgery

The transfrontal approach is now reserved for large pituitary tumours which are unresponsive to medical therapy, and which are either causing pressure effects or continuing to grow. Cure is rarely possible with large tumours and the main aim is decompression. If cure is achieved, it is nearly always at the cost of hypopituitarism. The main risks of transfrontal surgery are epilepsy and minor frontal lobe damage.

Transsphenoidal surgery

This is the treatment of choice — if the structure of the sphenoid bone allows it (see Fig. 2.1). The surgeon may be able to dissect out microadenomata and leave the surrounding normal gland intact. Alternatively, he or she may opt to remove as much pituitary tissue as possible at the expense of causing hypopituitarism. The transsphenoidal route is also suitable for decompression of very large tumours: removal of the tissue in the fossa allows suprasellar tumour to drop down. The main risk of transsphenoidal surgery is CSF rhinorrhoea. Temporary or permanent DI can complicate any form of pituitary operation.

Radiotherapy

External irradiation is widely used as adjunctive therapy. Treatment for 5 days a week for 4 weeks helps reduce tumours which are not curable by surgery. In the short term, radiotherapy makes people feel sick and ill. In the long term it can cause hypopituitarism.

Yttrium implantation

One or two centres have treated smaller tumours by implanting radioactive seeds of yttrium transsphenoidally.

Chapter 3
The Thyroid Gland

IODINE METABOLISM AND THYROID HORMONES

Iodide in the plasma is trapped by the thyroid and incorporated into the thyroid hormones, thyroxine (T_4) and triiodothyronine (T_3). T_4 and T_3 are essential for cell growth and development: the thyroid gland increases in size in puberty and in pregnancy. Thyroid hormones also help control the rate of cell metabolism throughout the body. Without T_4 and T_3 cell metabolism is slowed and growth is stunted.

Thyroid hormone synthesis is dependent on dietary iodide. Sea water is the main natural source of iodide, and until recently it was common for communities far from the sea to suffer as a result. In an attempt to trap more iodide, the thyroid gland enlarged, causing endemic goitre. The problem was also seen in limestone areas (e.g. Derbyshire neck). If the deficiency was gross, people would develop myxoedema and children would be stunted and cretinous. Nowadays, nearly all populations have their intake subsidized artificially. Iodine metabolism is summarized in Fig. 3.1.

ANATOMY

Development

The thyroid gland develops from the primordial pharynx (where it would have been in the best place to trap iodide in our fishy ancestors). It is recognizable in the first month of gestation when the fetus is only 4 mm in length. It develops from the floor of the mouth, between the first and second branchial arches, at the junction

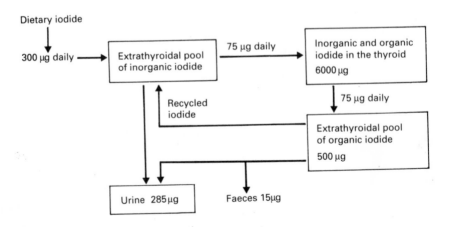

Fig. 3.1. Iodine metabolism.

of the anterior two-thirds and the posterior third of the tongue (stomadeum). It migrates caudally to take its position below the cricoid, on the front of the trachea.

It is joined by cells from the third and fourth arches, which form the lower and upper pairs of parathyroid glands respectively, as well as the parafollicular C-cells. The descent of the thyroid follows the thyroglossal duct, and part of this may persist as a thyroglossal cyst. The normal gland weighs 10–25 g and is composed of two lobes connected by an isthmus. Occasionally there is a central pyramidal lobe which represents the bottom of the thyroglossal duct (Figs 3.2, 3.3).

The main arterial supply to the gland is through superior and inferior thyroid arteries each side. These break up to form a rich plexus of arterioles: the blood supply to the thyroid is 4–6 ml min^{-1} g^{-1}, which is double that of the kidney. There is also a very rich nerve supply, with both postganglionic sympathetic and preganglionic parasympathetic fibres. It is thought that these control the blood supply, and this explains why people with enlarged thyroids often notice that the gland gets bigger at times of stress.

The fetal thyroid is functional before the 10th week, and the baby is independent of maternal thyroid hormones (which do not cross the placenta).

Anatomical relationships

The structures most closely related to the gland are shown in Fig. 3.2. The trachea and oesophagus may be deviated or compressed by any gross enlargement of the gland, while the parathyroids and the recurrent laryngeal nerve may be destroyed by a malignant tumour.

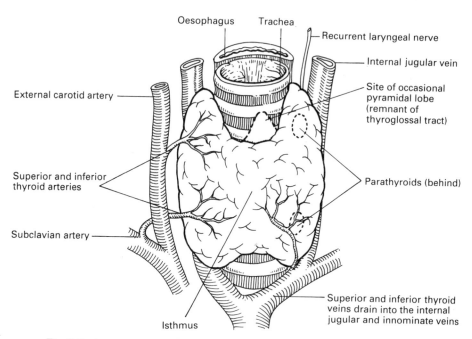

Fig. 3.2. Anatomical relations of the thyroid (anterior view).

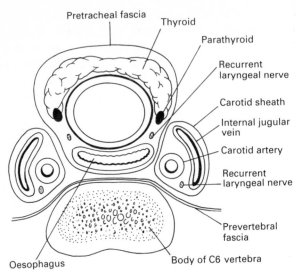

Fig. 3.3. Anatomical relations of the thyroid (cross-section).

Histology

The gland is composed of many follicles (acini), of up to 1 mm in diameter (see Fig. 1.7). Each follicle is lined by a layer of secretory cells and filled with colloid. T_4 and T_3 are made from iodotyrosines at the border between the colloid and the secretory cells, and are stored in the colloid, bound to thyroglobulin. A rich capillary network supplies the base of the secretory cells, and the capillaries are fenestrated, as in many endocrine glands.

THYROID HORMONES

The cells of the thyroid acinus synthesize thyroglobulin and mono- and diiodotyrosines, which are then transported to the colloid. While bound to thyroglobulin within the substance of the colloid, the iodotyrosines are converted to the iodothyronines T_3 and T_4. When T_3 and T_4 are secreted, they are hydrolysed from stored colloid before being secreted from the base of the acinar cell by pinocytosis into the capillary. T_4 is deiodinated in the liver, muscle and other tissues to T_3, or to its inactive isomer reverse T_3 (rT_3).

Control of thyroid hormone secretion

The thyroid is stimulated by pituitary thyroid-stimulating hormone (TSH). Secretion of pituitary TSH is itself under the control of hypothalamic thyrotrophin-releasing hormone (TRH), and is modulated by negative feedback by thyroid hormones. TSH enhances iodide uptake and both synthesis and release of T_4 and T_3. There is not much evidence that TSH is released in response to cold in humans, but there is a weak circannual rhythm, with very slightly higher levels of thyroid hormones in blood in winter. There is also a weak circadian rhythm, with T_4 and T_3 levels in blood being slightly higher in the morning.

Since thyroid hormones are essential for normal growth and development, and since the fetus is dependent on the supply of iodide (but not of thyroid hormones) by the mother, it is not surprising that the thyroid of the pregnant woman is under special control. TSH is largely suppressed in the first trimester, but the thyroid is stimulated by placental human chorionic gonadotrophin (hCG) which is phylogenetically related to TSH, and which has thyroid-stimulating activity. The gland enlarges to ensure that it traps sufficient iodide for both mother and baby. Transient thyroid dysfunction is very common in the months after delivery as the normal control of the maternal thyroid is re-established (see p. 67).

Thyroid hormones in blood

The total circulating concentration of T_4 (60–170 nmol litre^{-1} is about 50 times greater than that of T_3 (0.8–2.7 nmol litre^{-1}) 99.98% of T_4 and 99.7% of T_3 are protein-bound — to thyroid-binding globulin (TBG), albumin and prealbumin (now called transthyretin). All of circulating T_4, but only 20% of T_3, is secreted directly by the thyroid. The remaining T_3 in the circulation is derived by peripheral deiodination of T_4. This takes place in many tissues, but especially in liver and muscle (see Fig. 1.9). Since many cells possess the ability to convert T_4 to T_3, it is usually said that T_4 is a prohormone, and that it is T_3 which is the active substance. T_4 may also be deiodinated to the T_3 isomer, reverse T_3 (rT_3). Reverse T_3 is biologically inactive, and tissues produce either T_3 or rT_3 depending on requirements for cell growth and metabolism. Reverse T_3 is produced preferentially in a number of circumstances, and when it is, the measured concentration of T_3 in the blood is low (the 'low-T_3 sydrome', see Table 1.2). Since measured T_3 is so often low, it follows that a low T_3 concentration is not a reliable marker of hypothyroidism.

Thyroid function tests

The assessment of thyroid function by clinical examination is neither easy nor reliable, and all clinical management is dependent on measurement of thyroid function tests. These are of three types:

1 Measurement of effects of thyroid hormones on peripheral tissues, e.g. basal metabolic rate, hepatic enzyme induction and reflex relaxation time. These are imprecise and rarely used.

2 Measurement of iodine (or technetium) uptake by the thyroid gland. This is used more in the differential diagnosis of thyroid problems than in the assessment of overall thyroid function.

3 Measurement of thyroid hormone concentration in serum.

Measurement of thyroid hormone concentration in serum

T_4

This is the best overall guide to thyroid function. However, the measured concentration is very dependent on the concentrations of serum binding proteins (TBG, transthyrectin and albumin). Artificially high results will be found in pregnancy, oestrogen treatment (e.g. combined oral contraceptive), and in those with congenitally high levels of TBG. Congenitally low levels of TBG also occur, causing low T_4 concentrations.

Table 3.1. Thyroid function tests

Example 1
A 23-year-old woman complaining of being hot, sweaty, trembly and irritable, with staring eyes and 5 kg weight loss

T_4 268 nmol litre^{-1} (reference range 60–120)
T_3 4.8 nmol litre^{-1} (1.5–2.5)
TSH   < 0.1 mU litre^{-1} (0.8–4.5)

Diagnosis: Thyrotoxicosis

Example 2
A 56-year-old woman complaining of weight gain, feeling cold, dry skin and hair, constipation and a croaky voice

T_4 28 nmol litre^{-1}
T_3 1.8 nmol litre^{-1}
TSH   > 50 mU litre^{-1}

Diagnosis: Myxoedema

Example 3
A 28-year-old woman complains of irritability and difficulty sleeping, but no other relevant symptoms

T_4 185 nmol litre^{-1}
T_3 2.9 nmol litre^{-1}
TSH   2.8 mU litre^{-1}

Diagnosis: High level of T_4- and T_3-binding protein and normal TSH indicates that thyroid function is normal. Possibly congenital elevation of TBG, but more likely to be the contraceptive pill or pregnancy

T_3

A high T_3 is a good guide to overactivity of the thyroid, but a low T_3 is of no diagnostic value (see 'low-T_3 syndrome', Table 1.2).

TSH

TSH is now measured using highly sensitive and specific immunoassays: high results indicate primary thyroid failure; low results indicate thyroid overactivity (Table 3.1). Some laboratories use TSH as the main screening test. Sometimes, however, the TSH result may be misleading (Table 3.2). Serum TSH may be undetectable in early pregnancy, even though the woman has normal thyroid function.

Table 3.2. Circumstances in which TSH measurement may give misleading results

Assessment of people on T_4 treatment
People with treated thyrotoxicosis
People with hypothyroidism caused by pituitary TSH deficiency
Pregnancy

Other tests

Thyroid antibodies

Both hyperthyroidism and hypothyroidism are usually the result of autoimmune disease, with thyroid antibodies, respectively, stimulating or destroying the thyroid. In clinical practice it is usual to measure the thyroid antibodies which destroy the gland in hypothyroidism (antithyroglobulin and antimicrosomal antibodies), but the measurement of stimulating antibodies (thyroid-stimulating immunoglobulins, TSI) is difficult and expensive.

Ultrasound scan

This is used to determine whether a nodule in the gland is solid or cystic. If it is solid, there is an approximately 10% chance that it will be malignant. If cystic or partially cystic, the chances of malignancy are low.

Isotope scan

Uptake of radiolabelled technetium or iodine is used as follows:

1 Differential diagnosis of some forms of thyrotoxicosis: Graves' disease produces a uniform increase in uptake, whereas a toxic adenoma ('hot nodule') has localized uptake. When thyrotoxicosis is the result of subacute thyroiditis (see Table 3.3), uptake is reduced because the damaged cells are unable to trap iodide.

2 Diagnosis of dyshormonogenetic goitre: this is a rare familial condition characterized by inability of the gland to store and utilize iodide which has been trapped. There is increased uptake of isotope but it is washed out quickly because it is not incorporated into iodotyrosines (perchlorate discharge test).

The isotope scan is of no use in distinguishing between malignant and non-malignant causes of thyroid swelling.

Fine-needle aspiration cytology

If malignancy is suspected, cells can be aspirated under local anaesthesia and examined histologically. This technique is being used increasingly as a prelude, or alternative, to surgery.

Autoimmune processes and the thyroid gland

Population studies have found an overall prevalence of positive thyroid antibodies in 10–20% of the population. Clinically overt autoimmune thyroid disease affects only 2–4% overall, but is still extremely common. Thyroid diseases are 10 times more common in women than in men.

The predisposition to autoimmune thyroid disease is inherited, but the inheritance pattern is not simple. Susceptibility is linked to HLA major histocompatibility (MHC) genes, on chromosome 6. B8, DR3 and DR5 are variously associated with Graves' disease and hypothyroidism (with or without goitre), but many other associations have been described and it is likely that different genes are involved in different populations.

An environmental factor is required to trigger the onset of the autoimmune process. This factor — which may be a virus, or may be some other injury, or possibly even major psychological stress — stimulates the thyroid acinar cells to express their particular gene on the cell surface. The expression of this MHC antigen on the cell surface then stimulates local T-helper cells. These release lymphokines which in turn stimulate local B-lymphocytes to produce antibodies to the activated thyroid cells. These B-lymphocytes are all located within the thyroid gland itself (Fig. 3.4).

If the antibodies which are produced are destructive to the thyroid cells and their products (antimicrosomal, antithyroglobulin) then the person develops hypothyroidism, and this condition is called Hashimoto's thyroiditis (although the condition described by Hashimoto in 1912 was actually goitre with lymphocytic infiltration). If they are directed to the TSH receptor and, by binding to it, result in stimulation of the thyroid cell, the person develops thyrotoxicosis (Graves' disease). Other antibodies are thought to cause gland growth, and these may or may not be produced at the same time as other antibodies. The result is that some people with hypothyroidism and hyperthyroidism have big glands, whereas others do not. People with Graves' disease may also (uncommonly) produce antibodies which affect other tissues: the muscles of the orbit of the eye (thyroid eye disease, Graves' ophthalmopathy), the skin on the shins (pretibial myxoedema), and the subcutaneous tissues of the hands (acropachy). Activated B-lymphocytes may produce different antibodies at different times. The result is that people may go

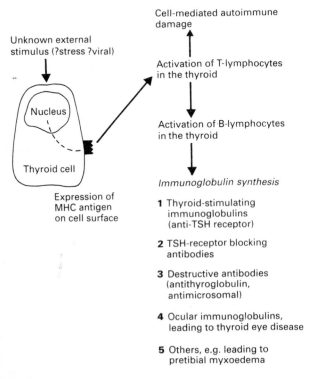

Fig. 3.4. Autoimmune processes and the thyroid.

from thyrotoxicosis to hypothyroidism, or even — very rarely — from hypo-thyroidism to thyrotoxicosis.

Post-partum thyroiditis

Approximately 20% of women have positive thyroid antimicrosomal antibodies in the early stages of pregnancy. The titre of antibodies falls as pregnancy advances, but rebounds in the first 3 months after delivery. Many of these women have transient abnormalities of thyroid function as a result (either overactive or under-active) and this is called post-partum thyroiditis. Despite being common, it is largely unrecognized in clinical practice. It is possible that some cases of post-natal depression (which affects approximately 15% of women in the first year after childbirth) may be attributable to transient changes in thyroid function, but this is unproven.

DISEASES OF THE THYROID

Diseases present with goitre (enlargement of the thyroid), hyperthyroidism (over-activity, thyrotoxicosis) or hypothyroidism (underactivity, myxoedema).

Goitre

There are a number of different reasons for the thyroid being enlarged.

Simple goitre

The thyroid enlarges normally in some people during puberty and pregnancy.

Iodine deficiency

Iodine deficiency causes hypothyroidism, with low circulating concentrations of T_4 and T_3. TSH increases because of reduced negative feedback. The thyroid enlarges under the influence of TSH.

Graves' disease and Hashimoto's thyroiditis

Some people with autoimmune disease have an enlarged thyroid, but some do not. There are three reasons for the gland enlarging:
1   Inflammation and lymphocytic infiltration.
2   Growth of thyroid cells by growth immunoglobulins.
3   In hypothyroidism, growth of surviving normal cells induced by TSH as the inflamed gland fails.

Subacute thyroiditis (De Quervain's disease)

This rare condition is thought to be viral, but may be autoimmune. The gland enlarges, becomes hard and is extremely painful. The person may be thyrotoxic in the acute phase due to the release of stored thyroid hormone, and can be rendered hypothyroid in the long term. Usually the condition settles completely in several weeks. Symptoms are rapidly relieved by oral corticosteroids. The main differen-tial diagnosis is from haemorrhage into a colloid cyst. An ultrasound scan will show no cyst, and an isotope uptake scan will show generalized reduced uptake of tracer.

Colloid goitre (multinodular goitre)

The colloid cysts distend such that they can be several millimetres, or even centimetres, across. The gland has either one palpable lump or several. They are firm, not hard. They are not painful (unless a haemorrhage occurs into one). The cysts will persist unless treated. There are three reasons for considering removal:

1 Cosmetic.
2 Exclusion of neoplasm.
3 Relieving pressure on adjacent structures.

Occasionally multinodular goitres become overactive (toxic nodular goitre), but the mechanism is not known.

Colloid nodules are common. They may be noticed as a swelling by the patient, or by a doctor or friend. The main fear is that the lump which has appeared is malignant. Although neoplasia tend to feel harder, malignancy cannot be excluded clinically. Demonstration of a 'cold nodule' with an isotope uptake scan is similarly useless, because both malignancy and colloid nodule will be 'cold' (i.e. will not concentrate tracer). Ultrasound examination will define whether the swelling is solid or cystic. If solid, there is a 10% chance that it is neoplastic. If cystic, it is very unlikely to be. Most centres would also now undertake fine-needle aspiration/biopsy cytology.

Dyshormonogenetic goitre

Dyshormonogenetic means that there is a congenital enzyme deficiency resulting in defective synthesis of thyroid hormones. There are several types, inherited as autosomal recessives, and all are rare. The person presents with a large fleshy thyroid in association with hypothyroidism. The diagnosis is clinched with the perchlorate discharge test which demonstrates that tracer taken up by the thyroid during an isotope uptake scan is washed out abnormally fast. When dyshormonogenesis is associated with congenital deafness, the condition is call Pendred's syndrome.

Neoplasia

The definition of neoplasia is difficult. The prevalence of histological neoplasia is very high: 4–8% of all post-mortems. None the less, clinical cancer occurs in only 0.8% of the population. Neoplasia can be classified as follows:

Benign, non-toxic adenoma

Adenoma formation is common in all endocrine glands. It will be solid on ultrasound, and the diagnosis will usually be made histologically after partial thyroidectomy.

Toxic adenoma, 'hot nodule'

Some adenomas cause thyrotoxicosis. The adenoma will concentrate tracer in an isotope uptake scan, while the surrounding gland is suppressed.

Lymphoma

Lymphomas are rare, but are more common in people who have autoimmune disease such as Hashimoto's thyroiditis. The other main cause of lymphomas is irradiation of the neck (e.g. radiotherapy to the neck in childhood).

Papillary carcinoma

Thyroid cancers typically arise in early- to mid-adult life, and 60–80% of them are papillary. They can be multiple. They are reasonably well differentiated, and cure by surgery and/or radioactive iodine is the rule rather than the exception. The 5-year survival rate for papillary carcinoma is 80%.

Follicular carcinoma

Follicular carcinomas occur in slightly older people — mid- to late-adult life. The prognosis is not quite so good because they tend to metastasize (to bone and lung). The 5-year survival rate is 60%.

Medullary carcinoma

Some 3–5% of thyroid cancers are medullary carcinomas. These are tumours of the parafollicular C-cells of the thyroid, which normally secrete calcitonin. Serum calcitonin concentrations may be high, but this is without obvious clinical or biochemical effect. However, they can also secrete other peptide hormones such as adrenocorticotrophic hormone (ACTH). Diarrhoea may occur but the mechanism is obscure. Medullary carcinomas tend to recur, and spread, locally, but are very slow-growing. They can arise as part of one of the multiple endocrine neoplasia (MEN) syndromes (see p. 105).

Anaplastic carcinoma

This uncommon condition occurs in the elderly — usually female. It is aggressive, spreads locally and is effectively incurable.

Other tumours

Because of its high blood supply, metastases often occur in the thyroid.

Treatment of thyroid tumours

Benign tumours are either left alone or treated by excision. Lymphomas are treated by chemotherapy. Papillary and follicular carcinomas are treated by a combination of total thyroidectomy and ablative dose(s) of radioactive iodine (4000 MBq ^{131}I). The person will require T_4 replacement therapy. Recurrences can be detected by interval scanning with tracer doses of ^{131}I since most retain the ability to trap iodide.

Thyrotoxicosis

Pathogenesis

The commonest cause of thyrotoxicosis is Graves' disease: stimulation of the TSH receptor by TSIs. Other causes are listed in Table 3.3.

Table 3.3. Causes of thyrotoxicosis

Common
Graves' disease (autoimmune)
Post-partum thyroiditis
Iatrogenic (or autogenic, 'factitious') overtreatment with T_3 or T_4

Quite common
Toxic multinodular goitre
Toxic adenoma (hot nodule)
Toxic phase of Hashimoto's thyroiditis (from gland destruction)

Rare
Toxic phase of subacute thyroiditis (from gland destruction)
Trophoblastic tumours:
    chorioncarcinoma and hydatidiform mole caused by excessive hCG

Extremely rare
TSH-secreting pituitary tumour

Drugs
Amiodarone

Clinical

The symptoms and signs result from:
1 The stimulatory effect of thyroid hormones on cell metabolism.
2 The synergism between thyroid hormones and the sympathetic nervous system.
3 Features of the underlying cause.
The person is trembly, irritable and nervous. They feel hot and sweaty, and lose weight despite usually having a good appetite. They may have diarrhoea, tachycardia or atrial fibrillation. Most people have retraction of the upper eyelids, causing lid lag and stare; the reason being the stimulation of catecholamine receptors on the levator palpebrae superioris.

Rarely, the presentation is unusual, with nausea or vomiting, and with apathy rather than nervous energy. Whether overactive or apathetic, the person may complain of tiredness caused by thyrotoxic myopathy. In Graves' disease the thyroid may be enlarged or not. If it is enlarged, it may be possible to hear the blood rushing through it by using a stethoscope (thyroid bruit). There may be other manifestations of the autoimmune process: thyroid eye disease, pretibial myxoedema, onycholysis (flaking of the nails) and acropachy (like clubbing).

Thyroid eye disease (Graves' ophthalmopathy)

Thyroid eye disease results from interaction between immunoglobulins and the external ocular muscles. These become inflamed and swell, later becoming fibrotic and adherent to surrounding tissues. The eye protrudes (proptosis) and the person may have double vision from asymmetrical ophthalmoplegia. The conjunctiva is oedematous (chemosis) and there may be periorbital oedema

(Fig. 3.5). Thyroid eye must be distinguished from simple lid lag and stare (caused by excessive circulating thyroid hormones): it pursues an unpredictable course and, unlike lid lag, does not improve as the thyrotoxicosis is corrected. Thyroid eye disease may be asymmetrical, and may even occur without the person being thyrotoxic. In such cases it may be necessary to exclude orbital tumours by computed tomography (CT) scanning.

Diagnosis of thyrotoxicosis

The diagnosis is confirmed by demonstrating elevation of serum T_3 and T_4 concentrations, with suppression of TSH. If T_3 and T_4 are elevated, but TSH is normal, the person is probably euthyroid with elevated TBG (usually from the contraceptive pill, hormone replacement therapy or pregnancy). If T_4 is elevated, T_3 is normal and TSH is suppressed, the person may be taking T_4 (factitious thyrotoxicosis). The tests which may be used in the diagnosis of cause are listed in Table 3.4.

If the thyroid is not palpable, or if there is a smooth symmetrical goitre, it is usually assumed that the person has Graves' disease.

T_3 toxicosis

Some people with thyrotoxicosis have elevation of T_3, but normal T_4 concentrations.

Treatment

There are three different types of treatment: tablets, surgery and radioactive iodine.

Tablets

Carbimazole is converted in the body to its active metabolite, methimazole. Propylthiouracil (PTU) has almost identical actions to carbimazole and is equally effective, but is less commonly used. Both block the uptake of iodide by the gland,

Table 3.4. Differential diagnosis of the common causes of thyrotoxicosis

Diagnosis	Thyroid	TFTs	Antibodies	Isotope uptake
Graves' disease	Impalpable or enlarged	High T_3 High T_4	Negative or weak positive	Increased
Toxic multinodular goitre	Nodular	High T_3 High T_4	Negative	Increased
Toxic Hashimoto's thyroiditis	Impalpable or enlarged	High T_3 High T_4	Strongly positive	Reduced
Toxic adenoma	Single nodule	High T_3 High T_4	Negative	Hot nodule
Iatrogenic or factitious	Impalpable	High T_4 but T_3 often normal	Negative	Reduced

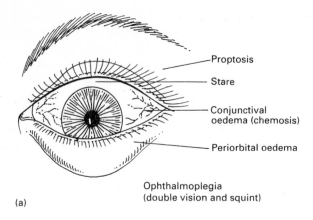

Proptosis

Stare

Conjunctival
oedema (chemosis)

Periorbital oedema

Ophthalmoplegia
(double vision and squint)

(a)

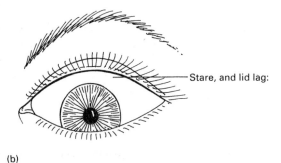

Stare, and lid lag:

(b)

Fig. 3.5. Eye signs in thyroid disease. (a) Cell-mediated and humoral autoimmune disease causing inflammatory infiltrate and swelling of the contents of the orbit; principally of the extraocular muscles. (b) Stare and lid lag. Rim of sclera is visible above top of iris either when looking straight ahead (stare), or when moving eye to look down (lid lag). It is caused by spasm of levator palpebrae superioris, and resolves when the thyrotoxicosis is treated.

and block its incorporation into iodotyrosines. Both drugs may cause skin rashes and, rarely (1 in 10 000 people treated), bone marrow suppression. The last is idiosyncratic and not dose-related, and is usually reversed when the drug is withdrawn. It is usual to start with larger doses (30–60 mg carbimazole daily; 300–600 mg PTU) and for these to be slowly reduced over the next few weeks. Some doctors continue with tablets for 18–24 months, but others withdraw them after just a few months to see if the condition relapses or not. Another approach is to treat for 18–24 months with high-dose carbimazole in association with replacement T_4.

If thyrotoxicosis relapses when tablets are withdrawn, there are two options: either long-term treatment with tablets, or definitive destructive treatment to the thyroid by surgery or radioactive iodine. Long-term tablet treatment may be chosen if the person is very old and frail, or if either of the other treatments is contraindicated or refused. In general, however, it is better to opt for definitive therapy.

Partial thyroidectomy

The advantage of partial thyroidectomy is that it reduces thyroid overactivity immediately, with a much-reduced chance of relapse. In good hands the operation carries minimal risk (specifically of damage to the recurrent laryngeal nerves, or to the parathyroids) and the wound heals quickly. Although it requires admission to hospital and a general anaesthetic, it may be cheaper in the long run by removing the need for multiple trips to outpatient clinics and blood tests. The main problem is that it is virtually impossible for the surgeon to judge the amount of gland which needs to be removed: 50% of cases are rendered euthyroid by the operation, 45% hypothyroid, and 5% will suffer recurrent thyrotoxicosis.

Radioactive iodine

Since 90% of ingested iodine is concentrated in the thyroid, 90% of an administered dose of radioactivity will end up there if it is attached to iodine. Treatment with oral ^{131}I has been widely used for over 40 years without obvious major side effects. It is simpler and cheaper than surgery, and is just as effective. Hitherto it has been reserved for the elderly, or at least for those who have completed their families. It is now being used increasingly in younger people.

Iodine

Iodine dissolved in potassium iodide (Lugol's iodine) is used by some surgeons prior to elective partial thyroidectomy. It will reduce thyroid hormone concentrations in previously untreated patients, but only for about 10 days. It is also thought to reduce the vascularity of the gland.

β-Blockers

Provided there is no contraindication (e.g. asthma, severe pre-existing heart failure), β-blockers are useful in thyrotoxicosis. They block the sympathetic manifestations of the disease and produce immediate symptomatic benefit. They also reduce peripheral conversion of T_4 to T_3. They are a helpful adjunct to definitive treatment.

Prognosis

Like many autoimmune diseases, Graves' disease comes and goes naturally. After a remission, the eventual chance of relapse is, however, very high: 50% relapse within 2 years and 80% within 25 years. For this reason it is important to keep these people under long-term surveillance. It is also important to monitor people who have been rendered euthyroid by surgery or radioactive iodine, because there is a risk of late hypothyroidism.

Thyroid storm

If a person with unrecognized thyrotoxicosis suffers major physical trauma (e.g.

accident, surgery under general anaesthesia, labour), there is a risk of thyroid storm. This is the term given to an acute, severe exacerbation of thyrotoxicosis, with tachycardia, hyperpyrexia and risk of circulatory collapse. It can be life-threatening in the elderly and infirm. If it occurs, it should be treated by:

1 Symptomatic treatment and support.
2 β-Blockers: propranolol 80 mg 6-hourly for an adult, or as necessary, provided there are no contraindications.
3 Carbimazole 15 mg four times daily (PTU 150 mg four times daily is preferred by some because it blocks conversion of T_4 to T_3).
4 Parenteral hydrocortisone 100 mg 6-hourly.

These treatments will need adjustment depending on individual circumstances and response.

Thyroid disease and pregnancy

Thyroid diseases commonly occur in young women, and hence often need to be managed through pregnancy and lactation. Moreover, there are a number of changes which take place in normal thyroid metabolism during gestation.

The normal thyroid in pregnancy

Because of the baby's requirements for iodine, the maternal thyroid enlarges in order to trap iodide more efficiently. Iodide crosses the placenta, but the mother's thyroid hormones do not. Control of the maternal thyroid is largely taken over by placental hCG (which has weak TSH-like activity, but circulates in large concentrations); TSH is often suppressed in the first trimester of normal pregnancy.

The immune system changes in pregnancy — presumably to avoid rejection of the genetically foreign fetus in the uterus. Approximately 20% of women develop positive antithyroid microsomal (not antithyroglobulin) antibodies in early pregnancy. Concentrations fall during the third trimester, but rebound after delivery, causing post-partum thyroiditis (see p. 67).

Diagnosis of thyroid disease in pregnancy

Diagnosis of thyroid status, especially of thyrotoxicosis, can be very difficult in pregnancy. Pregnant women normally have a goitre, and may have a tachycardia. Circulating T_3 and T_4 concentrations are normally increased because of the effect of oestrogens on TBG. Finally, TSH may normally be suppressed in the first trimester.

Management of Graves' disease in pregnancy

The mother must be kept euthyroid, by giving carbimazole or PTU in moderate doses (> 20 (> 200 for PTU) mg day^{-1}). However, these drugs cross the placenta and will make the baby hypothyroid if used in larger doses. Maternal Graves' disease — like all autoimmune conditions — tends to improve through pregnancy, and it is usually possible to reduce the tablets progressively. Most doctors stop antithyroid drugs altogether at 36–37 weeks, to prevent the danger of respiratory depression in the neonate, but this may not be possible if the mother's thyrotoxicosis is very active. If untreated at term, the mother is at risk of thyroid storm.

If the mother has very high concentrations of circulating TSIs, they can cross the placenta and make the baby thyrotoxic. This can be treated *in utero* by giving the mother antithyroid drugs. Thyrotoxicosis in the neonate will require treatment for only 2–3 months until maternal immunoglobulins are cleared.

Women taking antithyroid drugs should be allowed to breastfeed. Even though small amounts of the drugs are known to cross into breast milk (carbimazole more than PTU), it is thought that they are insufficient to have any significant effect on the baby — provided the mother is taking 20 mg (200 mg PTU) or less.

Management of hypothyroidism in pregnancy

Although some increase the dose of maternal T_4 in later pregnancy, most women require no adjustment of their treatment.

Trophoblastic tumours

Hydatidiform mole and chorioncarcinoma are benign and malignant tumours, respectively, of placental origin. They secrete hCG in high concentrations, and affected women are often thyrotoxic. They do not appear classically toxic, tending to be more apathetic, with nausea and vomiting.

Treatment of hydatidiform mole is evacuation of the uterus — with protective β-blocker therapy if necessary. Treatment of inoperable chorioncarcinoma is with chemotherapy, but small doses of antithyroid drugs may help nausea and vomiting.

Hyperemesis gravidarum

Some women develop very severe sickness in pregnancy — enough to require admission to hospital and intravenous fluids. In many such women there is biochemical evidence of thyrotoxicosis — thought to be induced by placental hCG — and treatment with low doses (5–10 mg) carbimazole can produce symptomatic benefit. Hyperemesis gravidarum usually improves after 16 weeks' gestation, when hCG levels start to fall.

Hypothyroidism

In hypothyroidism there is a generalized reduction in cell metabolism, with lowered basal metabolic rate and body temperature, mental slowing, apathy, dry skin, hair loss and constipation.

There is increased capillary escape of albumin, and the increase in extravascular albumin causes chronic oedema in the tissues. It is from this tendency that the alternative name of myxoedema (Greek *myxos* — tissue) is derived. Because of increased extravascular fluid the uterus is unable to contract efficiently, leading to menorrhagia. For similar reasons, hypothyroidism can also rarely present with isolated serous effusions — pleural, pericardial or peritoneal. Some hypothyroid people have symptoms of psychiatric disease — most commonly depression, but psychosis can occur (so-called 'myxoedema madness'). Hypothyroidism in childhood causes stunted growth and, if congenital and unrecognized, mental subnormality (cretinism).

Pathogenesis

There are two common causes: Hashimoto's thyroiditis and previous treatment for thyrotoxicosis with partial thyroidectomy or radioactive iodine. Even if Graves' disease has not been treated by surgery or radioactive iodine, the condition can evolve spontaneously into hypothyroidism with time. Similarly, hypothyroidism can follow subacute thyroiditis and post-partum thyroiditis. Other causes are listed in Table 3.5. The prevalence in Down's syndrome may be as high as 6%.

Clinical

The person with fully developed hypothyroidism has a pale and puffy face, thin and dry hair, flaking skin, a croaky voice, mental slowing, insensitivity to cold, weight gain and constipation. In addition, they may have menorrhagia, carpal tunnel syndrome, galactorrhoea, serous effusions and mental changes. On examination there is marked slowing of the reflex relaxation time (the speed with which the muscles relax after the knee, ankle or biceps jerks have been elicited).

In some people the signs are minimal and they are diagnosed by chance, or because they feel vaguely unwell or are troubled by increasing weight. Most doctors have a very low threshold for doing thyroid function tests, especially in the elderly.

Congenital hypothyroidism is endemic in iodine-deficient communities. If the baby is severely hypothyroid *in utero*, brain development will be defective and the

Table 3.5. Causes of hypothyroidism

Congenital
Congenital agenesis
Dyshormonogenetic goitre
Down's syndrome

Dietary
Iodine deficiency
Dietary goitrogens

Autoimmune
Hashimoto's thyroiditis
TSH-receptor blocking antibodies
Evolution of Graves' disease
Post-partum thyroiditis

Other
Subacute thyroiditis
Hypothalamic or pituitary disease
Addison's disease

Iatrogenic
Antithyroid drugs (carbimazole, PTU)
Other drugs (lithium, amiodarone)
Thyroidectomy
Radioactive iodine

child will be mentally subnormal (cretinous). Iodine deficiency is not the only cause of congenital hypothyroidism: approximately one baby in 4000 is born hypo-thyroid even in iodine-replete populations. The cause is usually sporadic agenesis of the thyroid gland. If the diagnosis is made early and replacement therapy started, the child may well not have any obvious physical or mental deficit. For this reason many countries undertake routine screening of thyroid function (measure-ment of TSH) at the end of the first week of life.

Diagnosis

The serum T_4 is low. A low T_3 is of no diagnostic value, because it can be low for other reasons ('low-T_3 syndrome'). If the hypothyroidism is caused by primary thyroid failure (as it usually is), the serum TSH is high (Fig. 3.6 and Table 3.1). Many laboratories rely on TSH assay for screening. TSH assay will be misleading, however, when the hypothyroidism is secondary to hypothalamic or pituitary disease and TSH deficiency (see Table 3.2).

In Hashimoto's thyroiditis the titre of antithyroid (antimicrosomal and anti-thyroglobulin) antibodies will be high.

Treatment

The daily replacement dose of T_4 is 50–200 µg for an adult. In clinically and biochemically mild cases, it is reasonable to start with 100 µg daily and adjust it depending on the blood levels. In more severe cases, and especially in the elderly and those with heart disease, it is safer to start with very low doses such as 25 µg daily. The dose should be doubled every 2 weeks or so, until the person is clinically and biochemically better.

Oral T_3 can be given, but is not often used. It has a shorter half-life and has to be taken two or three times daily. The standard 20 µg tablet causes a high peak of T_3, and the person may complain of flushing and palpitations.

Treatment of iatrogenic hypothyroidism

When treatment of thyrotoxicosis with surgery or radioactive iodine has rendered someone hypothyroid, and they have been started on replacement therapy with T_4, they may complain of persistent symptoms (lethargy, podginess) even when their serum T_4 is normal and their TSH is suppressed. The reason is not clear, but the consequence is that they tend to take a slightly higher dose of T_4 than appears necessary. The measured T_4 can therefore be slightly above the reference range in T_4-treated people, and the TSH is commonly suppressed. Intravenous T_3 (liothyronine) is available for the treatment of people who are unable to take tablets for any length of time. It can be given by a bolus injection of 5–20 µg.

Myxoedema coma

When hypothyroidism is so severe that the person is comatose, treatment needs to be undertaken with urgency and care. They need passive warming, cautious intravenous fluids and a nasogastric tube (oral fluids may be aspirated), and 5–10 µg bolus injections of T_3 (liothyronine) each 8–12 hours. The dose of T_3 can be increased depending on response; T_4 is substituted when they can swallow. It is

Primary hypothyroidism

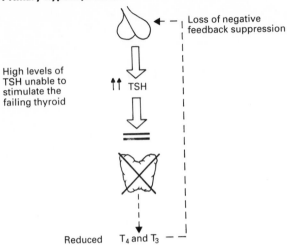

High levels of
TSH unable to
stimulate the
failing thyroid

Loss of negative
feedback suppression

↑↑ TSH

Reduced T_4 and T_3

Secondary hypothyroidism

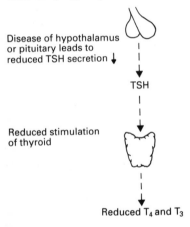

Disease of hypothalamus
or pituitary leads to
reduced TSH secretion ↓

TSH

Reduced stimulation
of thyroid

Reduced T_4 and T_3

Fig. 3.6. Serum TSH, T_4 and T_3 in primary and secondary hypothyroidism.

also usual to give parenteral hydrocortisone (50–100 mg 6-hourly). It is the
comatose patient with more severe long-standing hypothyroidism who is more
likely to develop psychosis. This 'myxoedema madness' may not be expressed
until they start to become more alert with replacement therapy.

Prognosis

The mortality rate in myxoedema coma is 50%. Life expectancy should be
otherwise normal in treated hypothyroidism.

Chapter 4
The Adrenal Gland and the Kidney

ANATOMY AND PHYSIOLOGY

Both the kidney and the cortex of the adrenal gland are derived from the urogenital ridge and are mesenchymal. The medulla of the adrenal is neuroectodermal. Although they are embryologically quite distinct, they are linked functionally and this explains their close anatomical relationship.

Kidney and adrenal cortex

Renin from the juxtaglomerular cells is necessary for secretion of aldosterone from the zona glomerulosa of the adrenal cortex.

Adrenal cortex and medulla

The enzyme which catalyses the formation of adrenaline from noradrenaline — phenylethanolamine-N-methyltransferase — is potentiated by glucocorticoids. These shared functions are directed towards preventing excessive salt and water loss and towards maintaining the effective circulation of blood.

The adrenal gland

The adrenal gland on each side weighs approximately 6 g, and lies above the kidney. The left adrenal is longer and thinner and reaches down the medial side of the upper pole of the kidney (Fig. 4.1). There is a capillary network which derives its arterial supply from the inferior mesenteric and renal arteries, as well as the aorta. The blood drains centripetally into the sinusoids (Fig. 4.2) and then through the medulla into the adrenal vein. The left adrenal vein drains into the left renal vein, and the right drains directly into the inferior vena cava.

Adrenal cortex

The cortex is divided into three zones: glomerulosa, fasciculata and reticularis (Fig. 4.2). The zona glomerulosa (Latin, *glomerulus*: blackberry) secretes predominantly mineralocorticoids. The fasciculata ('small ropes or cords' of cells) is the main source of glucocorticoids. The reticularis ('network' of cells) secretes glucocorticoids and androgens. However, the different zones are interchangeable: in response to adrenocorticotrophic hormone (ACTH) stimulation in Cushing's disease, the divisions become blurred. Moreover, zona glomerulosa cells in culture secrete glucocorticoids rather than mineralocorticoids.

Adrenal medulla

The secretory cells of the medulla are polyhedral and arranged in a loose meshwork of interconnecting cords. They are richly innervated by acetylcholine-

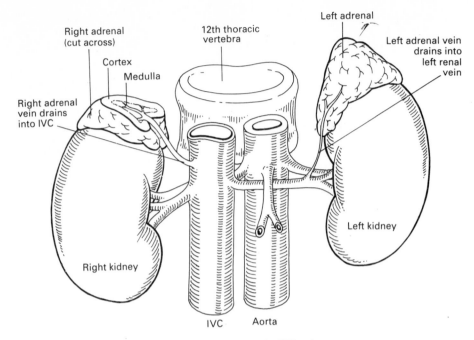

Fig. 4.1. Anatomical relations of the adrenal glands. IVC, inferior vena cava.

secreting preganglionic sympathetic fibres, and bathed in sinusoidal blood which drains centripetally from the cortex. Corticosteroids in this blood are essential for the formation of adrenaline from noradrenaline.

The secretory cells are called chromaffin cells, because they were shown (in 1900) to stain yellow–brown with chromium — hence 'affinity' for 'chromium'. Other chromaffin cells are distributed through the body in the liver, kidney, gonads, heart, carotid body, appendix and Peyer's patches of the small bowel. There are two types in the adrenal medulla: those which secrete noradrenaline, and those which secrete adrenaline. Both contain typical secretory granules — it is these that stain with chromium. The granules also contain a protein, chromogranin A, the function of which is unknown, as well as small quantities of leucine and methionine enkephalin. There is a third sort of cell — the pericyte — which is very closely related to the walls of capillaries and sinusoids, and which presumably modifies their function.

Hormones of the adrenal cortex

The adrenal cortex secretes steroids and these are divided into three groups, depending on their predominant biological actions: glucocorticoids, mineralocorticoids and sex steroids. The synthetic pathway of corticosteroids is given in Fig. 1.11. The main glucocorticoid in humans is cortisol, but in rodents it is corticosterone. The main mineralocorticoid in humans is aldosterone.

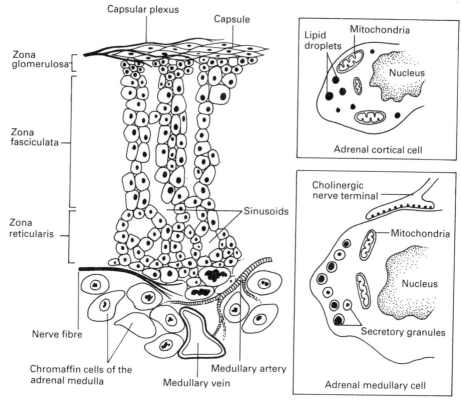

Fig. 4.2. Structure of the adrenal cortex and medulla.

Glucocorticoids

Actions

Glucocorticoids have many actions (Table 4.1). They also share some of the actions of mineralocorticoids. Glucocorticoids interact directly with X-protein to modify DNA transcription and the intracellular metabolism of arachidonic acid derivatives. Glucocorticoids are essential for life: an animal will die within days of bilateral adrenalectomy.

Effects of glucocorticoid excess

The effects of excessive glucocorticoid secretion (or excessive treatment with glucocorticoids) are listed in Table 4.2. Cushing's syndrome is caused by glucocorticoid excess.

Effects of glucocorticoid deficiency

The symptoms and signs of glucocorticoid deficiency are listed in Table 4.3.

Table 4.1. Main actions of glucocorticoids

Carbohydrate metabolism
Raise blood glucose by stimulation of glycogenolysis and gluconeogenesis

Protein metabolism
Increased breakdown, with overall negative nitrogen balance

Fat metabolism
Selective lipolysis, with loss of body fat in the limbs, but accumulation over the lower face and trunk

Suppression of inflammation
Reduced synthesis of prostacyclins; sequestration of eosinophils

Endocrine
Suppression of pituitary hormones: ACTH, LH, FSH, TSH, GH

Table 4.2. Effects of glucocorticoid excess (Cushing's syndrome)

Hyperglycaemia
From stimulation of gluconeogenesis and glycogenolysis

Negative nitrogen balance with protein loss
Osteoporosis, muscle wasting, reduced fibrogenesis, with thin skin and easy bruising

Salt and water retention
With tendency to congestive cardiac failure
Associated hypokalaemia

Reduced immune response
Increased susceptibility to infection

Abnormal fat metabolism
With increased fat deposition in central areas: face and trunk

Suppression of ACTH secretion

Neutrophilia

Mental effects
Including depression and confusion
Occasionally frank psychosis occurs

Mineralocorticoids

Actions

The predominant action of mineralocorticoids concerns the balance of salt, potassium and hydrogen ions: salt and water retention at the expense of K^+ and H^+. Mineralocorticoids also have weak glucocorticoid activity. Aldosterone is

Table 4.3. Effects of glucocorticoid deficiency

Increased sensitivity to insulin: tendency to hypoglycaemia
Reduced mobilization of peripheral protein and fat
Reduced gluconeogenesis
Inability to excrete a water load
Loss of salt and water: hyponatraemia and hyperkalaemia
Reduced neutrophils and increased eosinophils
Loss of feedback suppression of ACTH
Non-specific malaise, with fatiguability and gastrointestinal upset

thought to be responsible for 75% of the salt and water retaining effect, although the 24-hour secretion rate is much less than that of cortisol: 0.125 mg versus 20–25 mg.

Effects of mineralocorticoid excess

Excessive secretion of aldosterone results in salt and water retention, with loss of K^+ and H^+. This cases hypertension, with hypokalaemic alkalosis.

Effects of mineralocorticoid deficiency

Salt and water deficiency causes volume depletion with postural hypotension. There is associated hyperkalaemia and mild metabolic acidosis. In practice, the effects of mineralocorticoid deficiency are nearly always associated with those of glucocorticoid deficiency — Addison's disease.

Sex steroids

The adrenal cortex secretes androgens and oestrogens in both men and women. The biological significance of this, and the relationship between these sex steroids and those from the gonad, is not clear. Although the adrenals secrete testosterone in small amounts, they mainly produce weak androgens such as dehydroepiandrosterone sulphate (DHEAS) and androstenedione (see Fig. 1.11).

Effects of sex steroid excess

Androgens

The effects of androgen excess may be seen in women and children, but not in adult men. There are two causes: androgen-secreting tumours (p. 209), and congenital adrenal hyperplasias (pp. 92–6). Women may develop increased acne, with body and facial hair (hirsutism), frontal balding, increased muscle bulk, clitoromegaly and deepening voice (virilism). Children of both sexes enter a false puberty growth spurt. Boys develop signs of pseudopuberty (the testes remain small), and girls can develop clitoromegaly.

Oestrogens

The main effect of oestrogen excess in men is gynaecomastia. In premenopausal women it is menstrual disturbance with breakthrough bleeding.

Effects of sex steroid deficiency

There are none if gonadal function is intact. Children with Addison's disease go through a normal puberty.

Control of adrenocortical function

The control of secretion of glucocorticoids and sex steroids is different from the control of mineralocorticoids.

Glucocorticoids and sex steroids

Secretion is under the control of pituitary ACTH. If ACTH secretion is deficient, the person is cortisol-deficient. ACTH itself is under the predominant control of the hypothalamic releasing hormone CRH (corticotrophin-releasing hormone) and is released in three different ways:

1 Circadian rhythm: high in the early hours and morning, low in the evening.

2 Stress: physical and psychological stresses result in increased ACTH and cortisol secretion.

3 Negative feedback: ACTH secretion is suppressed by circulating glucocorticoids.

Mineralocorticoids

The main factor controlling aldosterone secretion is angiotensin II (AII). AII production is stimulated by the secretion of renin from the juxtaglomerular cells of the kidney (Fig. 4.3). However, other factors also act on the zona glomerulosa to increase aldosterone secretion:

1 Hyperkalaemia

2 Hyponatraemia

3 ACTH (to a small extent)

4 Other ACTH-related peptides

5 Prostaglandin E

Even though ACTH plays a small part, it is not significant in clinical practice. When a person is deficient in ACTH (from a pituitary tumour, for example), cortisol is low but aldosterone is normal.

Hormones of the adrenal medulla

Details of synthesis, secretion and clearance are given in Chapter 1. The effects of stimulation of α- and β-receptors by catecholamines are listed in Table 1.1.

The adrenal medulla secretes catecholamines (dopamine, noradrenaline and adrenaline) and peptides (enkephalins, somatostatin), often together. The main stimulus for hormone release appears to be stress, preparing the animal for 'fight or flight'. Thus the secretion of catecholamines will result in a differential supply of blood to brain, liver, muscles and kidney, and release glucose and fatty acids, which are then available as an energy source. However, the different roles of the different catecholamines and peptides is not clear, and neither is the relationship between the adrenal medulla and the rest of the sympathetic nervous system. The adrenal medulla is not essential, and an animal which has lost both is just as able to fight or be frightened as one which has not.

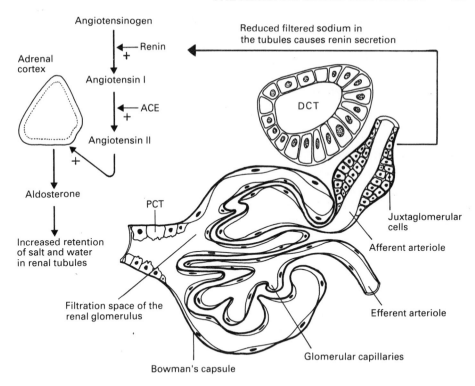

Fig. 4.3. Functional integration of the kidney and the adrenal cortex: the renin–angiotensin–aldosterone system. ACE, angiotensin-converting enzyme; DCT, distal convoluted tube; PCT, proximal convoluted tube.

Hormones and the kidney

The kidney has complex endocrine functions:

1 It secretes hormones, e.g. renin, erythropoietin (EPO).

2 It activates prohormones, e.g. 1,25-dihydroxycholecalciferol (1,25-OHCC).

3 It mediates the action of hormones, e.g. antidiuretic hormone (ADH), aldosterone, parathyroid hormone (PTH), atrial natriuretic factor (ANF).

4 It inactivates and clears hormones, e.g. prolactin, insulin.

Erythropoietin

The source of EPO in the kidney is not known, but it is probably the glomerulus. EPO has 166 amino acids (molecular weight 18 400 Da). It is released in response to falling tissue oxygen concentration, and its action is to stimulate red blood-cell production. Anaemia occurs in renal failure, partly because of EPO deficiency. Some renal adenocarcinomas secrete EPO to excess, resulting in polycythaemia.

Renin–angiotensin system

Renin is a glycoprotein of 347 amino acids (molecular weight 42 000 Da). Like many peptide hormones it is derived from prepro- and pro- forms. It is secreted into the blood stream from the juxtaglomerular cells of the afferent arteriole in response to:

1 Fall in ECF volume.
2 Fall in renal blood pressure.
3 Fall in the amount of sodium reaching the macula densa of the distal convoluted tubule (DCT).
4 Catecholamine stimulation.

All of these factors trigger renin release in order to increase renal conservation of sodium, and to maintain effective circulation of the blood. Information on the amount of sodium reaching the macula densa is possible because the DCT of each nephron loops back up to the renal cortex to bring the macula densa in close proximity to the juxtaglomerular apparatus.

Biological action

Renin is an enzyme which converts angiotensinogen to angiotensin I (AI). Angiotensinogen is a glycoprotein of molecular weight 52 000 Da, secreted by the liver. AI is converted to AII by angiotensin-converting enzyme (ACE, Fig. 4.3). ACE is widely distributed in body tissues, but particularly in the lung. AII is a potent octapeptide with two main actions:

1 It stimulates release of aldosterone from the adrenal cortex.
2 It sensitizes the smooth muscles of blood-vessel walls to the constrictor effect of noradrenaline: it raises blood pressure.

In addition, AII may play a role in the pituitary, modulating the secretion of anterior pituitary hormones.

Kallikreins

There are two broad groups of kallikreins: large-molecular-weight (107 000 Da) which circulate in plasma, and lower-molecular-weight (27 000–43 000 Da) which are present in organs (principally kidney, pancreas and salivary glands). They are proteases. In the kidney they are secreted from the renal tubule and have a pivotal role in regulating salt and water metabolism: they activate the renin–angiotensin system but they also antagonize it by releasing kinins (see below). Plasma kallikrein results in the generation of the potent vasodilator bradykinin (9 amino acids), while kidney kallikrein generates lysyl-bradykinin (10 amino acids).

Angiotensin-converting enzyme also helps modulate the balance between the renin–angiotensin system and the kinins: it activates AII, while it degrades kinins (ACE is a kininase) (Fig. 4.4).

Actions

Kallikrein catalyses the formation of renin from prorenin. It also catalyses the formation of kinins from kininogen. The actions of renin have been given above, but the actions of kinins are opposite; they:

1 Increase renal blood flow (RBF).
2 Increase the glomerular filtration rate (GFR).

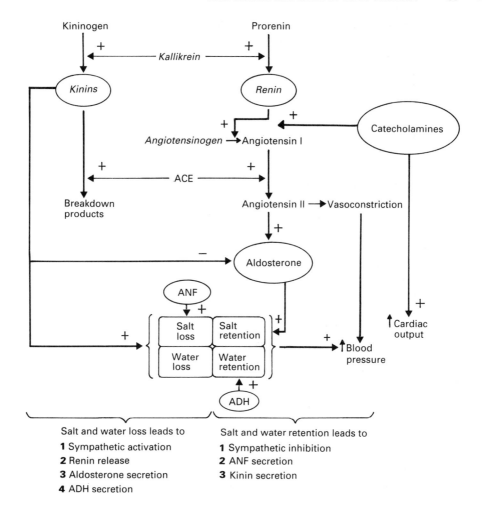

Fig. 4.4. Hormonal regulation of salt and water balance. ACE, angiotensin-converting enzyme; ADH, antidiuretic hormone; ANF, atrial natriuretic factor.

3   Increase renal loss of sodium and water.

4   Cause hypotension through vasodilatation.

Kinins also cause the synthesis of prostaglandins (principally PGA_2): they activate phospholipase, which liberates arachidonic acid (prostaglandin precursor, see p. 17) from membrane phospholipid. PGA_2 alters the renal tubular Na–K ATP-ase (adenosine triphosphatase) pump such that there is increased loss of sodium in the urine.

Atrial natriuretic factor (atriopeptin)

ANF is not secreted by the kidney but it acts on it. ANF represents a small family of peptides of which the main one has 31 amino acids, with a disulphide bridge. They are secreted by the muscle cells of the atrium of the heart in response to volume overload. They act on the kidney to increase salt and water loss.

Secretion

ANF is secreted in response to:
1   Atrial distension.
2   Any vasoconstrictor substance tending to cause a rise in blood pressure (e.g. noradrenaline, AII).
3   Sodium retention.
4   Tachycardia.

Actions

1   Increased GFR, leading to increased salt and water loss in urine.
2   Reduced renin secretion.
3   Reduced aldosterone secretion.
4   Antagonism of the vasoconstriction induced by AII.
The increase in GFR is achieved without an increase in RBF — presumably by causing constriction of the efferent arterioles of the renal glomerulus, with resultant increased filtration pressure. The reduction in aldosterone is partly the result of reduced renin, and partly due to a direct effect on the adrenal cortex.

Endocrine integration of balance of water and electrolytes

It will be obvious that many processes are integrated in the control of water and electrolyte balance. These processes have become progressively more complicated through evolution, with the need to maintain the integrity and the nutrition of large multicellular organisms such as humans, and especially of those which have left the sea to live on land. Not only does the body have to maintain overall hydration, it has to maintain an effective system of circulation. The endocrine processes are summarized in Fig. 4.4.

A warm-blooded, land-living animal has a persistent tendency to lose salt and water by evaporation. Hence most of the endocrine mechanisms are directed towards their conservation, with the renin–angiotensin–aldosterone system causing salt and water retention, while ADH conserves water alone. At the same time, the sympathetic nervous system and AII will ensure the maintenance of effective circulation by increasing cardiac output and increasing blood pressure through peripheral vasoconstriction.

None of these processes is allowed to proceed unchecked — volume overload and catastrophic hypertension would be the result if they were. Thus, there is a parallel system of counterregulation which operates to reduce blood pressure by vasodilatation (the kinins), and to increase salt and water excretion by the kidney (kinins and ANF). The attempts to conserve fluid and to excrete it are interconnected.

Thus, the heart and the kidney monitor the overall state of hydration of the body, and thereby help maintain an effective circulation to all cells. As the main need of cells is oxygen, it is not surprising that a hormone which regulates red-cell synthesis, EPO, is also secreted by the kidney.

ENDOCRINE DISORDERS OF THE ADRENAL GLAND AND KIDNEY

Hormonal causes of hypertension

There is no clear consensus on the part played by hormones in the pathogenesis of essential hypertension, although it is established that reduced intake of dietary salt is beneficial when the blood pressure is high. None the less, hormones can be implicated in a number of special circumstances.

Conn's syndrome

Primary hyperaldosteronism causes hypertension (with hypokalaemia) from excessive retention of salt and water.

Glucocorticoids

Glucocorticoids (either iatrogenic or in Cushing's syndrome) cause hypertension because of their weak mineralocorticoid effect. Glucocorticoids are also insulin antagonists and cause hyperinsulinaemia. This may also be implicated.

Oestrogens

The link between oestrogens and blood pressure is not understood, but there is an age-related increase in the prevalence of hypertension in women using oral contraceptives. The rise in blood pressure which occurs in some pregnant women (pregnancy-induced hypertension, pre-eclampsia) may be partly oestrogen-related, but its real causes remain obscure despite much study.

Renovascular hypertension

When one renal artery is critically narrowed, the kidney on that side receives and filters relatively little sodium. The consequence is that renin secretion rises, causing an elevation in AII, aldosterone and blood pressure. The cause of hypertension which accompanies renal failure (i.e. bilateral renal glomerular disease) is not known.

Phaeochromocytoma

Increased secretion of noradrenaline causes hypertension. Ethanol abuse is also associated with hypertension (and stroke), and this may be partly caused by the effect of ethanol on catecholamine secretion by the adrenal medulla.

Diseases of the adrenal cortex

Adrenocortical failure

Causes

Adrenocortical failure may be secondary (ACTH deficiency) or primary (disease of the adrenal gland). There are a number of different causes of deficiency of glucocorticoid and mineralocorticoid secretion (Table 4.4).

Table 4.4. Causes of adrenocortical deficiency

Pituitary ACTH deficiency (cortisol deficiency, but normal aldosterone)

Renin deficiency (very rare — aldosterone deficiency, but normal cortisol)

Primary disease of adrenal cortex:
   Addison's disease, caused by
     idiopathic atrophy/autoimmune disease
     tuberculosis
   Bilateral adrenalectomy
   Bilateral metastases
   Adrenal haemorrhage
   Haemochromatosis
   Adrenomyeloneuropathy
   Congenital adrenal hyperplasias:
     salt-losing
     non-salt losing

Drug-induced adrenocortical deficiency:
   Metyrapone
   opDDD (mitotane)
   Aminoglutethimide
   Ketoconazole
   Etomidate

Addison's disease

The cause of Addison's disease is usually autoimmune in the UK, even though circulating antiadrenal antibodies are demonstrable in only about 50% of cases. The glands have a lymphocytic infiltrate and become progressively atrophied. Tuberculosis (TB) is now a rare cause of Addison's disease in countries where antituberculous therapy is widely available (perhaps 5% in the UK), although worldwide it is the commonest cause. TB is suggested by a history of previous systemic tuberculous disease (a history of pulmonary TB alone is unhelpful), and by radiological evidence of calcification in the region of the adrenal glands. The finding of positive adrenal antibodies is strongly suggestive of an autoimmune aetiology.

The sex incidence of Addison's disease is equal. It can affect people of any age, but the diagnosis of Addison's in a child should raise the suspicion of either the rare HAM (hypoparathyroidism, Addison's disease, moniliasis) syndrome, or the rarer condition called adrenomyeloneuropathy or adrenoleukodystrophy (see below).

Haemochromatosis (very rare)

Haemochromatosis is an inborn error of iron transport which is more common in men (and much more common in other European countries, such as France, than it is in the UK). If untreated, the disease is complicated by deposition of iron in many tissues, but especially in the liver (leading to cirrhosis) and endocrine glands. The pancreas (diabetes) and pituitary (hypopituitarism) can also be involved.

Adrenomyeloneuropathy/adrenoleukodystrophy (extremely rare)
The two terms are used for the same X-linked condition — which is an extremely rare cause of adrenocortical failure. It is a disease characterized by the accumulation of abnormal long-chain fatty acids in the blood. This results in the defective function of cells which are heavily dependent on lipids for normal metabolism: the adrenal cortex, gonads, myelinated nerves. The disease is usually familial, affecting boys, and is characterized by the association of Addison's disease with progressive demyelination. It is untreatable and fatal within a few years.

Clinical

Adrenocortical failure is nearly always insidious in its onset, with weight loss, gastrointestinal upset and non-specific malaise. Glucocorticoid deficiency results in hypoglycaemia and reduced resistance to stress, while mineralocorticoid deficiency causes salt and water deficiency with postural hypotension. There is hyponatraemia, with a rise in plasma potassium and urea concentration. If the hyperkalaemia is extreme, the person may present with hyperkalaemic muscle weakness. With loss of negative feedback, ACTH concentration rises and this causes skin pigmentation.

The skin pigmentation of Addison's disease can be generalized, but can be localized to certain areas. These include the palmar creases, buccal mucosa, genitalia and nipples, recent operation scars, and light-exposed sites such as the face and the backs of the hands. If the adrenocortical deficiency is the result of ACTH deficiency, the tendency to hypotension and hyperkalaemia is less marked (because aldosterone secretion is normal), and there is no pigmentation.

Diagnosis

The diagnosis can be easy if the clinical picture is classic, but it can also be very difficult. Some suggestive biochemical features are listed below, but none is invariable and none is specific enough to be diagnostic on its own. The diagnosis is proved with the short Synacthen test.

Biochemical changes in Addison's disease
1 Hyponatraemia with hyperkalaemia.
2 Slight elevation in blood urea (haemoconcentration).
3 Low (< 250 nmol litre^{-1} at 0900 hours) or low–normal plasma cortisol in someone who is acutely ill.
4 High plasma ACTH (in primary adrenocortical disease).
5 Low plasma or urine aldosterone and high renin (in primary adrenocortical disease).
6 Relative neutropenia.
7 Eosinophilia.
8 Hypercalcaemia.
9 Low thyroxine (T_4) and high thyroid-stimulating hormone (TSH).

The short Synacthen test
Synacthen is the trade name of tetracosactrin, a synthetic peptide which com-

prises the first 24 amino acids of the ACTH molecule (39 amino acids). The short Synacthen test involves the intravenous or intramuscular injection of 250 µg (see Fig. 2.10). Failure of the plasma cortisol to rise above 600 nmol litre^{-1} indicates reduced adrenal cortical reserve. This test can be used for secondary as well as for primary adrenocortical failure.

Hypercalcaemia and adrenocortical failure

The pathogenesis of the hypercalcaemia is complex. It is partly the result of haemoconcentration, partly of increased osteolysis, and partly of altered renal handling of calcium in the face of sodium depletion. It responds rapidly to rehydration and treatment with corticosteroids.

Low T_4 and high TSH

These are the biochemical signs of primary failure of the thyroid. However, they may also be found in untreated Addison's disease. They should revert to normal when the hypoadrenalism is treated. If they do not, it indicates that the person has associated autoimmune thyroid disease which was not previously recognized: autoimmune Addison's, Hashimoto's disease and/or diabetes often coexist (Schmidt's syndrome).

Hypoadrenal (Addisonian) crisis

Although Addison's disease is insidious in its onset, many people present ultimately in crisis: they present as an emergency with signs of severe adrenocortical deficiency. They are profoundly ill, with hypotension, fever and prostration. The condition is fatal if untreated. The crisis may be precipitated by intercurrent illness. A rare cause of acute adrenocortical failure is haemorrhage into the gland complicating meningococcal septicaemia — Waterhouse–Friderichsen syndrome).

Treatment of Addisonian crisis

If acute Addison's disease is suspected, a sample should be taken for later cortisol assay and, if possible, a short Synacthen test done. However, treatment should not be withheld until the results are available. Emergency treatment consists of giving intravenous saline to replace salt and water deficiency, as well as hydrocortisone (cortisol). The hydrocortisone can be given in large parenteral doses if it is thought necessary (e.g. 100 mg 6-hourly), or can be given in more modest oral doses if the person is not acutely ill (e.g. 20 mg t.d.s). The normal maintenance dose for hydrocortisone is between 10 mg in the morning with 5 mg in the early evening, and 20 mg three times daily. Most people require 20 mg in the morning and 10 mg in the evening. If the person has aldosterone deficiency as well as cortisol deficiency, they require replacement with the synthetic mineralocorticoid fludrocortisone, in doses of 0.05 mg alternate days to 0.2 mg daily (see Table 4.5). If a person has tuberculous disease this should be treated with antituberculous chemotherapy. The prognosis for treated Addison's disease is excellent.

Congenital adrenal hyperplasia

The basic defect in congenital adrenal hyperplasia (CAH) is an inherited deficiency

Table 4.5. Corticosteroid replacement therapy

Hydrocortisone (i.e. cortisol)
Should be taken on waking and at tea-time. If taken later, it may cause wakefulness. 10 mg and 20 mg tablets

Cortisone acetate
Now rarely used because it requires conversion to cortisol in the body to be effective. 25 mg tablets

Prednisolone
Sometimes used instead of hydrocortisone but has no special advantages. 1 mg and 5 mg tablets

Dexamethasone
Like prednisolone it can be used but usually is not. 0.5 mg tablets

Fludrocortisone
Only used for mineralocorticoid replacement therapy. 0.1 mg tablets

Equivalent doses of glucocorticoids:
Hydrocortisone 20 mg
Cortisone 25 mg
Prednisolone 5 mg
Dexamethasone 0.5 mg

The synthetic glucocorticoid prednisolone has a double bond in the A ring. The synthetic mineralocorticoid fludrocortisone has a fluorine atom attached to C9.

of one of the enzymes necessary for cortisol synthesis. The glands become hyperplastic under the influence of ACTH in order to compensate for the lack of cortisol. The clinical picture is dependent on which enzyme is deficient, and on the severity of the defect.

Inheritance

The CAHs are relatively common autosomal recessive abnormalities, affecting between 1 in 2500 and 1 in 5000 live births in the UK. The siblings of an affected child have a 50% chance of being affected. The commonest defect by far involves the 21-hydroxylase enzyme (Fig. 4.5).

Clinical

If the enzyme defect is gross, the baby will die *in utero*. If the deficiency is partial the baby will survive, but will present in one of three ways:
1   The stress of birth and the neonatal period precipitates an Addisonian crisis (failure to thrive, hypoglycaemia).
2   A female infant is virilized.
3   The diagnosis is actively excluded because of a previously affected sibling.
Addisonian crisis occurs in the 'salt-losing' type. In this group the enzyme defect results in deficiency of aldosterone as well as of cortisol. This means that the infant is especially liable to salt and water depletion.

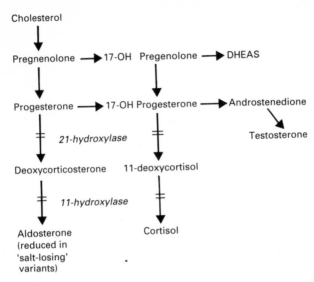

Fig. 4.5. Enzymes affected in CAH. Build-up of precursors proximal to the block (17-OH progesterone) leads to increased synthesis of androgens (DHEAS, androstenedione and testosterone).

Virilization occurs because of the build-up of cortisol precursors proximal to the enzyme block. When 17-OH pregnenolone and 17-OH progesterone accumulate, they are converted to androgens: androstenedione, DHEAS and testosterone (Fig. 4.6). The androgens in the circulation of the female fetus cause virilization of the external genitalia: clitoromegaly and varying degrees of fusion of the labia.

If there has been a previously affected sibling, the disease can be confirmed or excluded before birth by measuring the concentration of adrenal corticosteriods (usually 17-OH progesterone) in amniotic fluid obtained at amniocentesis.

Occasionally the diagnosis is missed at birth and the child will survive, provided the enzyme defect is not gross. The increase in circulating androgens causes a false puberty growth spurt when the child is at primary school, between the ages of 3 and 8. He or she will be big and strong, literally head and shoulders above their friends. However, the androgens then cause premature fusion of the epiphyses of the long bones, and final adult height is stunted. Women will remain muscular and virilized, with poor breast development and oligo- or amenorrhoea. Men will have normal secondary sexual characteristics. Both men and women will be pigmented because ACTH is elevated as a result of reduced negative feedback by corticosteroids on the pituitary. They will be at risk of Addisonian crisis if they develop any intercurrent illness.

Non-classic CAH

If the enzyme defect is very mild there may be no clinical suggestion of cortisol deficiency, even though the ACTH is high to overcome the block, and androgens

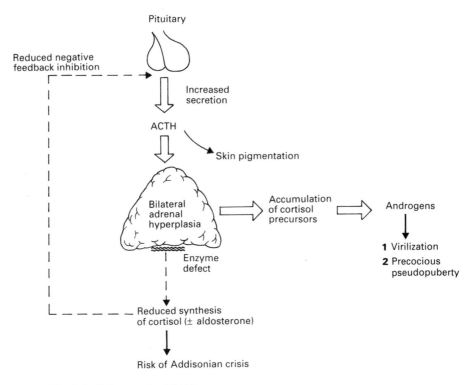

Fig. 4.6. Pathogenesis of CAHs.

are high as a result. Women with non-classic CAH (also called late-onset, or occult CAH) have acne, hirsutism or virilization. Affected men have no symptoms.

Diagnosis

Biochemical confirmation of the diagnosis is made by demonstrating any or all of:
1 Elevated plasma 17-OH progesterone.
2 Elevated plasma ACTH.
3 Elevated androgens.
4 Elevated urinary excretion products of adrenal androgens (pregnanetriol) — now rarely done.

A prenatal diagnosis can be made by measuring 17-OH progesterone (in 11- and 21-hydroxylase deficiencies) in amniotic fluid obtained at amniocentesis.

Treatment

The condition is analogous to Addison's disease: it is primarily a deficiency of cortisol, with or without deficiency also of aldosterone. Babies who are aldosterone-deficient as well as cortisol-deficient suffer salt and water loss in the neonatal period, and are called 'salt-losers'. Treatment is with glucocorticoid replacement therapy in an approximate dose of 5–10 mg m^{-2} day^{-1} hydrocortisone or equivalent, but judging the dose requires great skill. It is easy to establish that the child is given enough to suppress their markers of adrenal overactivity (17-OH progesterone, ACTH, etc.), but it is hard to make sure that they are not given too much. When a child is given excessive corticosteroids, final height will be stunted and they may also become cushingoid. Paediatricians monitor replacement therapy by keeping a very careful eye on the child's growth rate.

Once established on replacement therapy, the prognosis is generally the same as for Addison's disease. None the less, girls may require cosmetic surgery to correct the virilization of their genitalia. It is also said that girls who are salt-losers are likely to be relatively infertile.

Cushing's syndrome

Cushing's syndrome results from excessive glucocorticoids in the circulation. When it is non-iatrogenic (i.e. not caused by the administration of glucocorticoids), there is associated elevation of adrenal androgens. The actions of adrenal corticosteroids and effects of excessive secretion are summarized in Tables 4.1 and 4.2.

Cushing's syndrome can be a very difficult condition to diagnose and treat. As it is rare (fewer than five cases per million per year in the UK), it is best investigated and managed in specialist centres.

Causes

1 *Iatrogenic:* administration of glucocorticoids for medical reasons.

2 *Adrenal adenoma or carcinoma:* the cause in 10% of adults, but adrenal carcinoma is the commonest cause in children.

3 *ACTH-secreting pituitary tumour (Cushing's disease):* when Cushing's syndrome is caused by an ACTH-secreting pituitary adenoma, the condition is called Cushing's disease. This is the commonest cause in adults. The tumours are usually small and the pituitary fossa may not be expanded on skull X-ray (see also p. 51).

4 *ACTH secretion from a non-pituitary tumour:* this is called the ectopic ACTH syndrome. The commonest source of ectopic ACTH is small-cell anaplastic (oat cell) carcinoma of the lung.

Nodular hyperplasia of the adrenal cortex

There are rare cases of Cushing's in which ACTH secretion from a pituitary tumour causes nodular hyperplasia of the adrenals, and this can be complicated by one or more of the nodules becoming autonomous. This is analogous to the tertiary hyperparathyroidism of renal failure (see p. 229).

Intermittent or cyclical Cushing's disease

Some cases of pituitary-dependent Cushing's show a clear cyclical pattern, which makes diagnosis even more difficult — sometimes they have it and sometimes they do not. Presumably such intermittence is the result of hypothalamic dysfunction, with abnormal stimulation of ACTH release.

Alcohol-induced pseudo-Cushing's syndrome

This is a fashionable diagnosis, but the condition probably does not exist. Alcohol can certainly induce a body habitus very similar to that of Cushing's, but it is unlikely that it causes true glucocorticoid excess.

Clinical

The person develops central obesity, with a pendulous abdomen and a round red face (Fig. 4.7). There are increased supraclavicular fat pads and a 'buffalo hump' (a very non-specific sign) over the spinous processes of the lower cervical/upper thoracic vertebrae. The central obesity contrasts with gross thinning of the arms and legs due to muscle wasting. The overall habitus has been described as resembling a 'pear on matchsticks'. Loss of subcutaneous tissue results in easy bruising, with paper-thin skin. The skin of the trunk may be stretched, leaving livid deep-red 'striae distensae' (which are redder than the striae of pregnancy, and broader than the thin striae which some adolescents develop when they increase rapidly in height or weight). Because of an increased susceptibility to infection the person may have skin infections, especially tinea or monilia.

Mental changes are very common in Cushing's syndrome. Depression affects over 50%, and a few are frankly psychotic. Some have a characteristic mental state, with fretful uncertainty and insecurity. The depression and frank psychosis may respond well when the condition is successfully treated, but the other features can persist and be a frustrating feature of long-term management.

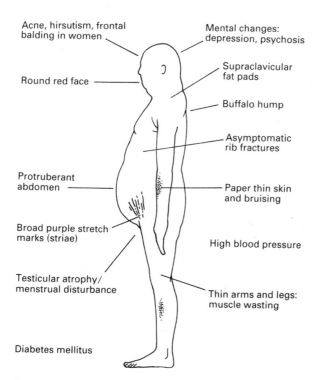

Fig. 4.7. Clinical features of Cushing's syndrome.

Increased secretion of androgens may result in hirsutism, or male-pattern baldness, with or without menstrual irregularity. This does not occur if the condition is drug-induced because synthetic corticosteroids have very little androgenic activity.

If Cushing's syndrome is caused by excessive ACTH secretion, there may be associated skin pigmentation. The areas affected are the same as those in Addison's disease, but the degree of pigmentation is not usually marked unless the person has ectopic ACTH secretion or Nelson's syndrome and the ACTH concentrations are particularly high. Some increase in pigmentation occurs in simple obesity, especially around the axillary folds and areas subjected to pressure by clothing. Since hypertension, glucose intolerance, hirsutism, menstrual irregularity and depression are common accompaniments of simple obesity, the clinical diagnosis of Cushing's syndrome can sometimes be difficult.

Further examination and investigation may reveal osteoporosis, with a tendency to spontaneous fractures which are often painless: a person may limp into the clinic with a spontaneous fracture of a tibia or pubic ramus, or may be found on routine chest X-ray to have fractured ribs. These fractures are characteristically surrounded by exuberant callus — presumably because they are painless and the area is not immobilized, allowing shredded periosteum to lay down new bone over a larger area.

The blood pressure is elevated because of an increase in mineralocorticoid activity, and the ankles are often swollen. This ankle swelling is usually ascribed to increased salt and water retention, but this cannot be the reason because ankle swelling is not a feature of pure mineralocorticoid excess (Conn's syndrome — see below). It probably results from the effect of glucocorticoids on the capillary escape of albumin.

Glucocorticoid excess may cause glucose intolerance or frank diabetes. Mineralocorticoid excess may cause hypokalaemia, but the plasma potassium concentration is unlikely to be < 3.0 mmol litre^{-1} unless:

1   the person has received diuretics for ankle swelling, hypertension or both, or
2   the Cushing's syndrome is the result of ectopic ACTH secretion.

It is not known why people with ectopic ACTH secretion are more likely to have hypokalaemia than people with other types of Cushing's syndrome.

Diagnosis

The clinical suspicion has to be confirmed by demonstrating excessive and inappropriate amounts of circulating corticosteroids. The overnight dexamethasone test (the plasma cortisol should be < 60 nmol litre^{-1} at 0900 hours after 1 mg dexamethasone at midnight) is the easiest way of excluding Cushing's syndrome in people in whom the clinical suspicion is not high. The test has false negatives — high sensitivity but not very high specificity.

Twenty-four hour urine cortisol excretion is also very sensitive, but highish levels may be encountered in obesity, depression or stress. The test with the highest specificity (few false positives) is the hypoglycaemia stress test.

Note that it is not necessary to measure ACTH (which is difficult and expensive to do) to diagnose Cushing's syndrome. Assay of ACTH is necessary only for determining the *cause* of the Cushing's — which is best undertaken in specialist centres.

Diagnosis of the cause of Cushing's syndrome

An adrenal tumour will be suspected in a child (adrenal carcinoma is the commonest cause in children), or if there is other evidence of an adrenal mass. Ectopic ACTH secretion will be suspected if there is an obvious non-pituitary tumour, in those with very high plasma and urinary cortisol, and in those with deep pigmentation. The tests which help define the cause of Cushing's syndrome include:

1 *Plasma potassium concentration:* concentrations less than 3.0 mmol litre^{-1} (in people not taking diuretics) are strongly suggestive of ectopic ACTH secretion.

2 *ACTH concentration:* this will be undetectable in people with adrenal tumours.

3 *High-dose dexamethasone (8 mg day^{-1} for 48 hours):* those with ectopic ACTH secretion are unlikely to suppress at all, whereas those with pituitary Cushing's retain some partial feedback control.

4 *Pituitary-dedicated computed tomography (CT) scan:* this is helpful if it shows a macroadenoma, but large pituitary tumours are unusual in Cushing's disease.

5 *CRH test:* intravenous injection of 100 µg of the hypothalamic hormone CRH will result in an exaggerated rise in plasma ACTH in pituitary-dependent Cushing's disease.

Treatment

1 *Treatment of cause:* removal of an adrenal or pituitary tumour, or a source of ectopic ACTH, may be curative.

2 *Pituitary adenomas:* these are usually best treated by transsphenoidal selective adenomectomy. Initial cure rate is high, but there is a relapse rate of 20–40%. Large tumours may be approached transfrontally. A pituitary adenoma may also be treated by external irradiation, or by implantation of radioactive seeds of yttrium into the pituitary fossa. Sometimes ACTH secretion can be reduced by drugs (e.g. cyproheptadine, bromocriptine) but the response is usually only partial.

3 *Bilateral adrenalectomy:* if the person has ACTH-dependent Cushing's, but the actual source of ACTH is not clear, or if previous specific therapy has been unsuccessful, the manifestations of the disease can be reversed by removing both adrenal glands. There is a small risk in pituitary-dependent disease that bilateral adrenalectomy removes some feedback suppression of the pituitary tumour, allowing it to become big and aggressive. This is called Nelson's syndrome; it can be very difficult to treat (see p. 53).

4 *Drugs to reduce adrenal steroid secretion:* drugs which reduce cortisol secretion can be used as an adjunct to definitive therapy (preoperative preparation with drugs reduces complications), or they can be used when other therapy has failed, e.g. in adrenal carcinoma. The prognosis in adrenal carcinoma is very poor, and it is nearly always impossible to resect the tumour completely. Survival beyond 2 years from diagnosis is very exceptional.

Metyrapone (250 mg b.d.–750 mg t.d.s) and aminoglutethimide (250 mg b.d.– 500 mg t.d.s.) cause reversible inhibition of cortisol synthesis. On the other hand, opDDD (mitotane) reduces steroid secretion because it is adrenolytic (destroys adrenal cells). Other drugs (e.g. ketoconazole, etomidate) also have actions on the adrenal cortex, but they are not used routinely for the treatment of Cushing's.

Conn's syndrome: primary hyperaldosteronism

Cause

Excess aldosterone secretion is nearly always the result of adrenocortical disease: hyperaldosteronism secondary to a renin-secreting tumour is exceptionally rare (Fig. 4.8).

The zona glomerulosa, which secretes the aldosterone, may contain an adenoma, or be hyperplastic, or both. The occurrence of diffuse hyperplasia suggests that the zona glomerulosa is being stimulated by an outside factor. If so, that factor is not known. Nor is it known why adenomas and hyperplasia may coexist in the same gland.

Carcinoma of the zona glomerulosa is extremely rare.

Clinical

Hyperaldosteronism causes hypertension in association with marked hypokalaemia (plasma $K^+ < 3.0$ mmol litre^{-1}). Any person with high blood pressure and hypokalaemia, especially a young person with no relevant family history, should have the condition excluded. Occasionally, however, severe hypertension can induce secondary hypokalaemia in its own right, by causing renal tubular damage. Overall, the commonest cause of hypokalaemia in hypertensives is diuretic treatment.

Diagnosis

Conn's syndrome is confirmed by demonstrating high plasma or urinary aldosterone in association with suppressed renin. An adenoma may be demonstrable on CT scan. If it is, selective catheterization of the adrenal veins may confirm that aldosterone is coming from the enlarged gland, but not from the contralateral one. High concentrations of aldosterone in both adrenal veins suggests that there is hyperplasia of both zonae glomerulosae.

An alternative way of demonstrating whether overactivity is unilateral or bilateral is by performing an iodocholesterol adrenal isotope scan. Dynamic tests of aldosterone release (change in plasma aldosterone concentration with posture, or change following administration of Synacthen) do not differentiate reliably between adenoma and hyperplasia.

Treatment

The effects of the hyperaldosteronism can be reversed by administering the aldosterone antagonist spironolactone in high doses (up to 400 mg orally each day). In some people, and especially in those with evidence of hyperplasia, long-term treatment with spironolactone is the treatment of choice. Spironolac-

Primary hyperaldosteronism

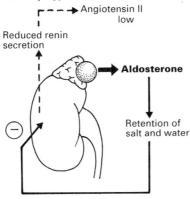

Secondary hyperaldosteronism

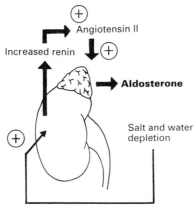

Fig. 4.8. Primary and secondary hyperaldosteronism. Primary hyperaldosteronism (Conn's syndrome) is caused by an adenoma of the zona glomerulosa, hyperplasia, or both. Secondary hyperaldosteronism — any cause of low blood volume (haemorrhage, dehydration, nephrotic syndrome) leads to increased renin and aldosterone secretion. Primary renin-secreting tumours also cause secondary hyperaldosteronism, but are very rare.

tone is oestrogenic, however, and may suppress libido and potency in men. If an adrenal adenoma can be defined, and if selective catheterization or iodocholesterol scan confirms that the contralateral gland is not also overactive, then unilateral adrenalectomy is usually the treatment of choice.

Endocrine manifestations of renal disease

Endocrine abnormalities occur in renal failure, in renal tubular disease and with certain renal tumours.

Renal failure

Many hormones exert their actions on the kidney (e.g. glucocorticoids, mineralcorticoids, arginine vasopressin (AVP), atrial natriuretic factor (ANF), and many are cleared there (e.g. insulin, growth hormone (GH), prolactin). The kidney also activates some hormones (1,25-OHCC), and secretes some (e.g. renin, erythropoietin). There are thus multiple endocrine defects in renal failure.

Calcium metabolism

Calcium will fall because of reduced 1-hydroxylation of vitamin D. The tendency to hypocalcaemia is worsened by phosphate retention caused by glomerular failure (renal rickets). This causes secondary hyperparathyroidism and increased mobilization of calcium from bones (renal osteodystrophy). There may be associated hypomagnesaemia. Patients may be treated with agents to reduce phosphate absorption, as well as with oral 1-hydroxylated vitamin D (alfacalcidol or calcitriol).

Hyperprolactinaemia

Approximately one-third of patients with established renal failure have hyperprolactinaemia. This can contribute to general malaise, and can also account for impotence or amenorrhoea. Some respond well to treatment with bromocriptine. Raised serum GH concentrations are not clinically significant.

Hyperinsulinaemia

There is reduced clearance of insulin in renal failure. Insulin-dependent diabetics with renal failure suffer recurrent hypoglycaemia unless the dose of injected insulin is reduced.

Hypertension and renal failure

Hypertension commonly complicates renal disease. In renovascular disease (renal artery stenosis) the hypertension is caused by increased renin secretion. In glomerular failure salt and water retention is an important factor, but in most cases the cause of the hypertension is unknown.

Reduced erythropoietin

EPO is a 166-amino acid peptide secreted by the kidney in response to reduced oxygen availability. It acts on the bone marrow to increase red-cell synthesis. Reduced secretion of EPO is the main cause of the normochromic, normocytic anaemia which complicates renal failure. Synthetic EPO is available for treatment and works well, but is not routinely given because of its cost.

Renal tubular disorders

Any cause of renal tubular dysfunction may cause hypokalaemia (with kaluria) or nephrogenic (ADH-resistant) diabetes insipidus (DI). In addition there are a number of rare congenital disorders of renal tubular function.

DIDMOAD syndrome

The association of nephrogenic DI with diabetes mellitus (DM), optic atrophy (OA) and deafness (D).

Bartter's syndrome

Bartter's syndrome is a rare congenital disorder in which there is hyperaldosteronism and hypokalaemia, but normotension. There is an unspecified defect of prostaglandin synthesis in the kidney which causes abnormal chloride reabsorption in the loop of Henle. There are other variable tubular defects, causing DI, hyponatraemia and hypokalaemia through renal potassium loss. There is hyperreninaemia and secondary hyperaldosteronism. The condition can be treated by giving potassium supplements, with or without prostaglandin synthesis inhibitors such as indomethacin.

Renal tubular acidosis

Classic type

There is an abnormality of the distal tubule which results in excessive reabsorption of H^+ ions. There is hyperchloraemic acidosis of the blood, with inappropriately alkaline urine. There is variable loss of sodium, calcium and potassium by the kidney. It responds well to treatment with bicarbonate.

Proximal type

There is an abnormality of the proximal tubule which results in defective reabsorption of bicarbonate. There is hyperchloraemic acidosis, with alkaline urine. It may be associated with other renal tubular defects (aminoaciduria, glycosuria — Fanconi's syndrome), and nephrocalcinosis (from hypercalciuria) is common.

Renal tumours

Renin-secreting tumours

Renin may be secreted by benign haemangiopericytomas (tumours of cells of the juxtaglomerular apparatus). This causes secondary hyperaldosteronism with hypertension (often severe) and hypokalaemia. It is differentiated from Conn's syndrome by demonstrating that concentrations of renin and AII are high, rather than low.

Renin may also be secreted by Wilms' tumours (nephroblastomas).

EPO-secreting tumours

EPO may be secreted by adenocarcinomas of the kidney, as well as by rare haemangioblastomas of the cerebellum and elsewhere. The von Hippel–Lindau syndrome is characterized by multiple haemangioblastomas (cerebellum, retina, visceral organs) and is autosomal-dominant, but most haemangioblastomas are non-hereditary. Excessive EPO causes polycythaemia.

Diseases of the adrenal medulla

No apparent harm comes from underfunction of the adrenal medulla. The only clinically significant diseases of the adrenal medulla result from tumour formation. There are three types of tumour and all are extremely rare.

Neuroblastoma

Neuroblastomas occur in children. There are about 80 cases each year in the UK, which makes it one of the commonest childhood cancers. Ninety per cent are endocrinologically active, but the tumour is so malignant that children tend to present with metastases rather than with the effects of increased catecholamine secretion. Treatment is by attempted excision, combined with radiotherapy/chemotherapy.

Ganglioneuroma

This is even more rare than the neuroblastoma. It tends to occur in rather older children or young adults. It is malignant, but not as aggressive as neuroblastoma.

Phaeochromocytoma

Clinical

The incidence of phaeochromocytoma is approximately the same as that of neuroblastoma. It presents in adulthood with hypertension, which may be either sustained or paroxysmal. It is a very uncommon cause of hypertension, and there is no point in screening for it in all people with high blood pressure: only in those with suggestive associated symptoms and signs — unexplained fear, panic attacks, tachycardia, hyperglycaemia — or in those with a positive family history.

Ten per cent are malignant, 10% are bilateral (in familial syndromes — see below — 40% are bilateral) and 10% are extra-adrenal.

Undiagnosed phaeochromocytomas present a considerable hazard if the person undergoes abdominal surgery or goes into labour: death can occur from hypertensive crisis.

Diagnosis

The diagnosis is made by demonstrating elevated concentrations of catecholamines in blood or urine. Assays for plasma catecholamines are highly specific, but not widely available. Urinary catecholamines are adequate for most purposes, although mild elevations are rarely significant. False elevation of plasma concentrations may be found in those who are stressed, or who are being treated with vasodilators or monoamine oxidase (MAO) inhibitors. False elevation of urinary concentrations may occur for a number of reasons (Table 4.6).

Table 4.6. Factors interfering with measurement of plasma and urinary catecholamines

Biological
Physical or mental stress
Diet: coffee, bananas, nuts
  cheese may lead to high plasma levels because of its
  tyrosine content
Drugs: MAO inhibitors, vasodilators

Artefactual
Interference with urinary assay method:
  methyldopa, labetalol, tetracycline, chlorpromazine

Localization of phaeochromocytomas can be made using CT or MRI (magnetic resonance imaging) scanning, or by scanning with radioactively labelled MIBG (meta-iodobenzylguanidine). Angiography can also be used, after suitable preparation with α- and β-blockers (see below).

Treatment

Treatment is by excision wherever possible. Prior to surgery the patient should have the effects of the catecholamines nullified by administration of the α-blocker phenoxybenzamine (10 mg t.d.s.) and the β-blocker propranolol (80 mg t.d.s., or more) for 3 days. If it is not possible to resect the tumour, the condition can be treated by administering α-methylparatyrosine, which acts as a false transmitter.

Multiple endocrine neoplasia and familial syndromes

Multiple endocrine neoplasia (MEN) is the name given to the association of two or more different hormone-secreting tumours in the same person. Phaeochromocytoma is a feature of some, but not all, of them. They may be sporadic or familial. Inherited forms are usually autosomal-dominant, but with incomplete penetrance.

MEN type I (Werner's syndrome)

Affected people may have tumours of the parathyroid (90%), pancreatic islets (80%) and pituitary (60%). Pancreatic tumours are often gastrinomas (Zollinger–Ellison syndrome).

MEN type II (Sipple's syndrome)

Phaeochromocytoma occurs in most, with associated medullary carcinoma of the thyroid and hyperparathyroidism. The hyperparathyroidism is usually the result of hyperplasia rather than adenoma. Inheritance of familial forms is linked with the centromeric portion of chromosome 10.

Type IIb

These patients have neurofibromas of the face causing distortion of the lips and jaw, as well as the endocrine features of Sipple's syndrome. They tend to be tall and thin (marfanoid).

MEN type IIIa (von Recklinghausen's disease)

Phaeochromocytoma, medullary carcinoma of the thyroid, multiple neuromas of the skin, subcutaneous tissue and mucosa, meningiomas, gliomas and orbital tumours.

MEN type IIIb (von Hippel–Lindau syndrome)

Phaeochromocytoma, islet-cell tumours, haemangioblastomas of the cerebellum and orbit, renal adenocarcinoma. The haemangioblastomas secrete EPO, causing polycythaemia.

Medullary carcinoma of the thyroid

This is a tumour of the calcitonin-secreting parafollicular C-cells of the thyroid. These cells are thought to have a different embryological origin from the other cells of the thyroid gland — possibly neural crest rather than endoderm. This explains the association of medullary carcinoma with other tumours of neural tissue, as in von Recklinghausen's disease. The condition is the rarest of all forms of thyroid carcinoma and is frequently familial.

Calcitonin is a 32-amino acid peptide which inhibits bone resorption. In many species it tends to lower serum calcium, but its physiological function in humans is not known. People with medullary carcinoma of the thyroid usually have high circulating concentrations of calcitonin but their serum calcium is normal. In most cases the only symptom or sign of the disease is the presence of a lump in the thyroid gland, but diarrhoea sometimes occurs. Because of the frequency of familial cases, it is usual to undertake family screening when a case is identified. Apart from clinical examination, screening involves measuring serum calcitonin (basally or after stimulation with either calcium or pentagastrin) and exclusion of phaeochromocytoma.

Medullary carcinomas of the thyroid may secrete hormones other than calcitonin.

The only treatment is excision of the tumour. Unresectable tumours are resistant to both radiotherapy and chemotherapy, but tend to grow only slowly.

Chapter 5
Endocrinological Aspects of Malignancy

ECTOPIC HORMONE SECRETION

Some tumours secrete hormones which are not normally secreted by the gland or tissue which contains the tumour. This is called ectopic hormone secretion. It is probable that it occurs because the tumour is derived from multipotential stem cells which differentiate abnormally. It is also possible that the gland or tissue *does* normally synthesize the hormone, even though it is not usually thought to, and hence it is not ectopic at all. A good example of this is the commonest form of ectopic hormone secretion of all: adrenocorticotrophic hormone (ACTH) secretion by small-cell anaplastic (oat cell) lung cancer. Although it was not realized when ectopic ACTH secretion by lung cancer was first described, it is now known that ACTH is normally produced by cells of the bronchial mucosa, and it is these cells which are stimulated by cigarette smoke and other irritants to form small-cell anaplastic carcinoma. The ACTH content of the lungs of cigarette smokers is much higher than in non-smokers.

Ectopic ACTH syndrome

Ectopic ACTH secretion will cause Cushing's syndrome, provided that the levels of ACTH are high enough for long enough. This can occur with slowly growing tumours of the lung, as well as rare tumours of the thymus, thyroid, adrenal medullae, pancreas and gonads. The commonest cause, however, is small-cell anaplastic (oat cell) lung cancer. In many cases the cancer is so aggressive that it does not allow the classic features of Cushing's syndrome to develop: the person loses weight, rather than gains it. In such people the only signs may be deep pigmentation (from high ACTH concentrations) and hypokalaemia. For reasons which are not clear, the plasma potassium is much lower in ectopic ACTH than in other types of Cushing's syndrome.

HYPERCALCAEMIA OF MALIGNANCY

There are a number of different reasons why people with cancers can develop hypercalcaemia. These include the secretion of one or more substances which stimulate osteoclastic resorption of bone — osteoclast-activating factors — or which have parathyroid hormone (PTH)-like activity, such as PTHrp (PTH-related peptide).

HORMONE DEPENDENCE OF TUMOURS

Tumours of the breast and prostate are particularly sensitive to circulating concentrations of sex steroids. Meningiomas have been shown to have large numbers of progesterone receptors, and may respond to new progesterone-blocking agents such as mifepristone.

HORMONE PRODUCTION BY TUMOURS

If hormone production by tumours of the endocrine glands is excluded, as well as ectopic hormone secretion, there remains a small group of (relatively rare) tumours which are endocrinologically active.

Teratomas

Teratomas of the ovary and testis contain elements which resemble trophoblastic tissue, both histologically and functionally. Like normal placenta, they can secrete human chorionic gonadotrophin (hCG).

Trophoblastic tumours

Hydatidiform moles and chorioncarcinomas secret hCG. The hCG can cause thyrotoxicosis.

Adenocarcinoma of the kidney

EPO is normally secreted by the kidney, and adenocarcinomas can secrete erythropoietin to excess. They can therefore be associated with polycythaemia.

Inappropriate ADH secretion

Inappropriate secretion of antidiuretic hormone (ADH) by the hypothalamus can occur with many different conditions, including lung cancers. However, in a minority of cases the lung cancer appears to cause the condition by secreting ADH directly.

ENDOCRINOLOGICAL CONSEQUENCES OF THE TREATMENT OF MALIGNANCY

Treatment of tumours by either radiotherapy or chemotherapy can have endo-crinological consequences.

Cranial irradiation

Cranial irradiation can cause hypopituitarism.

Gonadal irradiation or systemic chemotherapy

The likely consequence in both men and women is sterility, because the effect of these treatments is most marked on rapidly dividing cells, such as spermatogonia. There is also a theoretical risk that, if a man or a woman has a child following treatment with significant doses of ionizing radiation, there will be an increased incidence of fetal abnormalities.

Irradiation to the thyroid

There is an increased risk of thyroid malignancy, particularly of lymphoma, following external irradiation.

Chapter 6
Gut Hormones — Hormones of the Enteroinsular Axis

The first hormone ever described, in 1902, was a gut hormone: secretin. Gut hormones fall into two broad types: those secreted by cells scattered diffusely through the gut, and those secreted by cells gathered into recognizable clusters — as in the islets of Langerhans in the pancreas. Although more is known of the latter type, it has been difficult to apply classic techniques to investigate their physiological and pathological role more fully. One particular problem is that the hormones act both locally, on adjacent cells (paracrine action), as well as by being carried to more distant cells by the blood stream (endocrine action). Moreover, it is into the portal circulation that they tend to be secreted, rather than the systemic circulation, and this has made it difficult to study changes in blood concentrations. With the important exception of insulin, little is known of their physiological role and of the part they play in disease. Apart from diabetes mellitus, recognized diseases are rare and are confined to tumours of the cells secreting gut hormones.

Insulin, glucagon, somatostatin, cholecystokinin (CCK), and gastric inhibitory peptide (GIP) are all true hormones in that they are carried by the blood stream to their target sites. There are also a number of other 'candidate hormones' which probably exert their main actions on adjacent cells, acting as paracrine rather than endocrine transmitters. The true hormones probably have additional paracrine actions.

Many of the gut hormones are phylogenetically and structurally related. For instance, secretin, GIP, vasoactive intestinal polypeptide (VIP) and glucagon all have structural similarities and are said to belong to the 'secretin family'. Some of the main gut hormones, and their designated cells of origin, are listed in Table 6.1

Some gut hormones (e.g. somatostatin, cholecystokinin, neurotensin) are also found widely distributed throughout the central nervous system (CNS), where they act as neurotransmitters.

Secretin (27 amino acids)
Most secretin cells are found in the duodenum and upper jejunum. The hormone is released in response to gastric acid. It stimulates water and bicarbonate secretion by the exocrine pancreas, and also inhibits gastric acid secretion.

Gastrin (17 amino acids)
Secretion of this short polypeptide by gastric cells is stimulated by food, distension, falling gastric pH, the vagus and other factors. Its release causes gastric acid secretion and contraction of the oesophageal sphincter, allowing effective intragastric digestion of food. It probably also has an action in maintaining the growth of gastrointestinal cells. It is curious that gastrin-secreting tumours (gastrinomas)

Table 6.1. Pancreatic and gut hormones and their cells of origin

Tissue	Cell classification	Hormone/peptide
Pancreas	B	Insulin
	A	Glucagon
	D	Somatostatin
	D	VIP
	PP	Pancreatic polypeptide
Stomach	G	Gastrin
	A	Enteroglucagon
	D	Somatostatin
	P	Bombesin
Duodenum	S	Secretin
	K	GIP
	EC	Motilin (+ 5HT)
	I	CCK
	P	Bombesin
Colon	D1	VIP
	L	Enteroglucagon

are not found in the stomach — which is the normal site of gastrin-secreting cells — but in the pancreas.

CCK

CCK exists in multiple forms, including CCK 33, CCK 41 and CCK 58 — the numbers indicate the polypeptide chain length. Like secretin, CCK is secreted mainly by the upper small bowel, in response to food as well as vagal stimulation. Its main actions include pancreatic enzyme secretion and gallbladder contraction.

GIP (43 amino acids)

GIP is secreted by cells in the lower part of the duodenum in response to intraluminal glucose (fast phase) and fat (slow phase). It was originally named gastric inhibitory peptide because it was shown to inhibit gastric motility. It is now thought, however, that its main action is to augment pancreatic insulin secretion in response to hyperglycaemia. Its new name, glucose-dependent insulinotropic peptide, was devised to fit its original acronym. It has a number of other actions, including reducing the secretion of gastrin and pepsin.

VIP (29 amino acids)

VIP is present in cells throughout the whole small bowel, and is released in response to gut distension by food. It stimulates contraction of the smooth muscle of the gut wall, but also has a number of other actions including the stimulation of pancreatic exocrine secretion and insulin secretion, and inhibition of gastrin and gastric acid. It may act as an overall modulator of intestinal motility, blood flow, secretion and absorption.

Like most gut hormones, VIP is also found in many other — non-gastrointestinal — sites, where its functions are different. In particular, VIP is found in association with the smooth muscle of blood-vessel walls and of the genital tract.

Glucagon (29 amino acids)

Glucagon is derived from proglucagon (called glicentin). The glucagon in the pancreas and in the intestinal wall ('enteroglucagon') are structurally identical (29 amino acids), although enteroglucagon may also be present in smaller fragments. Glucagon causes vasodilatation in mucosal and submucosal vessels, but has a number of metabolic effects as well, especially the stimulation of glycogenolysis and gluconeogenesis — resulting in a rise in blood sugar. The main actions of glucagon are opposite to those of insulin.

Pancreatic polypeptide (36 amino acids)

Pancreatic polypeptide (PP) is secreted by the pancreas in response to vagal and sympathetic stimulation, as well as to CCK. It is structurally related to other peptide transmitters, neuropeptide Y (NPY), and peptide YY. It is often found in tumours secreting other gut hormones. Its physiological and pathological functions are unknown.

Somatostatin (14 amino acids)

The occurrence and function of hypothalamic somatostatin has been described above. However, the peptide is widely distributed throughout the body, and presumably has different actions in different sites. It is secreted by the D-cells of the pancreas and results in reduced secretion of insulin, as well as CCK, GIP and VIP. It is secreted also by cells throughout the small intestine.

Motilin (22 amino acids)

Motilin is structurally unrelated to any of the other gut hormones. Its release from EC-cells in the duodenum is affected by the absence, rather than the presence, of food. It is thought to control gastrointestinal motility during fasting.

Bombesin (14 amino acids)

Bombesin was identified in the skin of frogs (*Bombina* spp.). Its main action in humans is the stimulation of gastrin release.

Insulin

Structure

Insulin is secreted by the β-cells of the islets of Langerhans. It is composed of two peptide chains linked by disulphide bridges (A-chain 21 amino acids, B-chain 30 amino acids — see Fig. 1.2). Because diabetes is essentially a disease of insulin deficiency, and because it is so common, insulin has been studied more than any of the other pancreatic and gut hormones.

Table 6.2. Some factors affecting insulin secretion

Stimulation of secretion
Blood glucose
Glucagon
Amino acids: lysine, leucine
Growth hormone
Parasympathetic innervation (vagus)
Gut hormones: enteroglucagon, secretin, CCK
Other hormones: ACTH, TSH

Inhibition of secretion
Hypocalcaemia
Noradrenaline
Somatostatin

Secretion

Insulin secretion is secreted spontaneously in 13-minute cycles from isolated islet cells, but *in vivo* the most important stimulus to secretion is glucose. Secretion is integrated with that of glucagon, because the two hormones have essentially opposite actions on carbohydrate metabolism. Many different nervous and hormonal factors modulate insulin secretion (Table 6.2). The details of their functional integration is not known, but there is a two-phase insulin response to any stimulus, the fast phase representing the release of stored peptide.

Target cell interaction

Insulin binds to specific receptors on target sites, and the insulin–receptor complex is taken into the cell. The complex is broken down within cytoplasmic lysosomes, stimulating a cellular response. The second messenger mechanism is unknown.

Biological actions

The main biological actions of insulin are shown in Table 6.3.

Effects of insulin excess

The commonest cause of insulin excess is the over-treatment of diabetes. How-

Table 6.3. Actions of insulin

Target organ	Action of insulin
Liver	Glycogen synthesis
	Prevention of ketone formation
Muscle	Glucose uptake
	Glycogen synthesis
Fat	Glucose uptake
	Inhibits lipase and lipolysis

ever, insulin may be secreted to excess by insulin-secreting tumours, insulinomas, and in nesidioblastosis.

The result of acute insulin excess is hypoglycaemia. Chronic hyperinsulinism causes lipogenesis, with fatty infiltration of the liver and obesity. Acute administration of insulin with glucose is used in the emergency treatment of hyperkalaemia: glucose and insulin drive potassium into the cells.

Effects of insulin deficiency — diabetes mellitus

Partial

Relative insulin deficiency results in hyperglycaemia, as in Type II (non-insulin dependent) diabetes.

Total

When there is no effective circulating insulin, the body is unable to utilize glucose as an energy source and relies instead on acetoacetate and hydroxybutyrate (ketone bodies) generated by lipolysis. Ketone bodies are acidic, and when they accumulate in excess the patient develops ketoacidosis. Untreated ketoacidosis is fatal within hours or days. Total insulin deficiency is the hallmark of Type I (insulin-dependent, ketosis-prone) diabetes.

HORMONE-SECRETING TUMOURS OF THE PANCREAS

Vipoma

Vipomas are tumours of the pancreas which secrete VIP. They present with torrential watery diarrhoea, colicky abdominal pain, dehydration and, sometimes, flushing. The tumours are often malignant but may be completely removable if found early. If incurable, symptoms may be helped — for a while — with strepto-zotocin (which destroys pancreatic endocrine cells), 5-fluorouracil (a less specific cytotoxic) or a somatostatin analogue (somatostatin and its analogues reduce the secretion of many hormones, including those of the endocrine pancreas). VIP may also be secreted by ganglioneuroblastomas.

Glucagonoma

Glucagon-secreting tumours of the pancreas are usually tumours of the A-cells of the islets of Langerhans, but enteroglucagonomas also occur. The condition presents in a characteristic way, with rash, diabetes, diarrhoea and venous thromboses. The rash is described as spreading, necrotizing, bullous and eryth-ematous. The diabetes occurs because glucagon is an insulin antagonist. The mechanism for the other symptoms is not known.

The majority of these tumours have metastasized by the time of diagnosis, but symptoms may respond to treatment with streptozotocin, 5-fluorouracil, and somatostatin analogues.

Gastrinoma (Zollinger–Ellison syndrome)

These are gastrin-secreting tumours of the endocrine pancreas (rarely primary tumours of the gut). Unlike vipomas and glucagonomas, gastrinomas tend to pursue an indolent course. Even people with tumours which have metastasized at diagnosis may survive for several years. Complete tumour removal is rarely possible and so is rarely attempted. Streptozotocin and 5-fluorouracil have been used, but the most useful treatment is with drugs that reduce gastric acid secretion, such as H_2-receptor antagonists and potassium/hydrogen ATPase inhibitors. The main feature of gastrinomas is severe recurrent peptic ulceration, which is the result of increased gastric acid secretion induced by gastrin. Thirty per cent of sporadic gastrinomas are associated with parathyroid tumours. Hypercalcaemia normally stimulates gastrin secretion, and so it is possible (but unproven) that in some cases the gastrinoma is caused by the hyperparathyroidism.

Insulinoma

Insulinomas are the most common of pancreatic endocrine tumours. This is because insulin-secreting cells are the most common cells in the islets of Langerhans. Insulinomas present, predictably, with hypoglycaemia induced by the inappropriate secretion of insulin. The history of attacks may be short, and the person is referred to hospital with little doubt about the diagnosis. More usually, the person suffers with recurrent attacks of abnormal sensation or behaviour for many years before hypoglycaemia is suspected. In such cases the diagnosis can be difficult to prove (see Hypoglycaemia, below).

Ten per cent of insulinomas are malignant, and 10% are multiple. They are removed surgically, if possible, but it is also usually possible to manage people with benign insulinomas for many years, using the drug diazoxide. Diazoxide is related to the thiazide diuretics and reduces insulin secretion. Its use is complicated by sodium retention and a tendency to congestive cardiac failure. Thiazide diuretics also inhibit insulin secretion to some extent, which is why their use can exacerbate or precipitate diabetes mellitus.

Nesidioblastosis

Hyperinsulinaemia may rarely result from diffuse hypertrophy of the islets of Langerhans. It is one cause of neonatal hypoglycaemia, but it can also occur in adults.

Somatostatinoma

Somatostatin normally reduces insulin secretion, gastric acid secretion, intestinal absorption and gallbladder secretion. When a somatostatinoma causes excessive somatostatin secretion, the results are predictable — diabetes, hypochlorhydria, steatorrhoea, weight loss and gallstones. Somatostatinomas are usually pancreatic, but can occur in the bowel. The diagnosis is confirmed by demonstrating high circulating levels of somatostatin. Some also secrete calcitonin. The only effective treatment is attempted total excision, but it is usually unsuccessful.

HYPOGLYCAEMIA

Clinical

The common symptoms and signs of hypoglycaemia are summarized in Table 6.4. They have two basic causes:

1 Neuroglycopenia.
2 Catecholamine release.

The brain is absolutely dependent on glucose as an energy source. When blood glucose is reduced, the person may become confused, behave abnormally, or lapse into coma. In older people with some cerebrovascular disease, hypoglycaemia may present with lateralizing CNS signs like a stroke. Others may develop *grand mal* fits, and this is also a characteristic feature of hypoglycaemia in babies.

The second set of symptoms and signs results from the massive outpouring of catecholamines which occurs in response to hypoglycaemia. The body releases them in an effort to elevate blood glucose by glycogenolysis and gluconeogenesis.

Causes

The commonest cause of hypoglycaemia is the inappropriate administration of insulin, or of sulphonylurea drugs which release pancreatic insulin. This is usually accidental, but it may be wilful or manipulative — especially in adolescent diabetics and medical and paramedical professionals who have diabetes. Accidental hypoglycaemia caused by sulphonylurea drugs is so common that the diagnosis should always be suspected when an older diabetic treated with one of these drugs suffers any paroxysmal attacks (headache, sweating, weakness, etc.), or symptoms suggesting a transient ischaemic attack, or unconsciousness.

The other main cause of hypoglycaemia is starvation. Many women can become technically hypoglycaemic (venous blood sugar < 2.2 mmol litre^{-1}) after simply fasting for 24 hours or more. Starvation-induced hypoglycaemia is more likely if people already have depleted glycogen stores, or if they take alcohol. Alcohol impairs gluconeogenesis and will induce hypoglycaemia in anyone who is starving and who has exhausted his or her glycogen reserves.

Insulinoma is a rare cause of hypoglycaemia, as are adrenocortical failure, nesidioblastosis and retroperitoneal tumours (Table 6.5). Reactive hypoglycaemia

Table 6.4. Clinical features of hypoglycaemia

Neuroglycopenia
Hunger
Dizziness or confusion
Lateralizing neurological signs
Coma

Catecholamines
Anxiety, fear, agitation
Sweating
Pallor
Tachycardia, palpitations

Table 6.5. Causes of hypoglycaemia

Common
Normal variant
Alcohol-induced reduction in gluconeogenesis
Administration of insulin or oral hypoglycaemic agents
Reactive hypoglycaemia
Liver disease (defective glycogenolysis and gluconeogenesis)

Uncommon
Hypoadrenalism
Insulinoma
Nesidioblastosis
Tumour-associated hypoglycaemia

---

results when large amounts of insulin are released in response to a glucose load. This occurs typically after gastric surgery, but may also occur in otherwise normal people who eat a lot of sweet foods, and in some people with incipient diabetes. There are multiple causes of hypoglycaemia in neonates.

Tumour-associated hypoglycaemia

Rare tumours such as retroperitoneal sarcoma can present with hypoglycaemia. Such tumours secrete an insulin-like peptide, IGF_2, with hypoglycaemic activity.

Diagnosis of hypoglycaemia

When someone is identified as being truly hypoglycaemic (blood glucose < 2.2 mmol litre^{-1}), and if there is no obvious reason such as insulin or sulphonyl-urea administration, it is essential to take a sample for the laboratory for later analysis of both glucose *and* insulin. This should be done before treatment is given, if at all possible. If insulin is detectable in the blood of someone who is hypogly-caemic, they have either received a drug to make them hypoglycaemic, or they have an insulinoma. This is the only easy, reliable way to make the latter diagnosis.

CARCINOID TUMOURS AND THE CARCINOID SYNDROME

Carcinoid tumours are tumours which arise in the gastrointestinal tract and in tissues of gut origin (notably the lung, thymus and pancreas). They are tumours of cells which are normally endocrinologically active. The tumours were called 'carcinoid' because they resembled carcinomas histologically, but appeared to behave in a benign fashion. In fact, carcinoid tumours may be benign or malignant, and may grow slowly or extremely fast. Small-cell anaplastic (oat cell) carcinoma of the lung is a highly malignant form of carcinoid tumour.

Carcinoid tumours arising in derivatives of the embryological foregut (lung, thymus, pancreas) typically produce peptide hormones, whereas tumours in the lower gut tend to produce amines, particularly 5-hydroxytryptamine (5-HT), but also tryptophan and kallikrein (which catalyses the formation of bradykinin). It follows that carcinoid tumours of foregut derivatives present with excessive secretion of peptides such as ACTH: i.e. with Cushing's syndrome, whereas

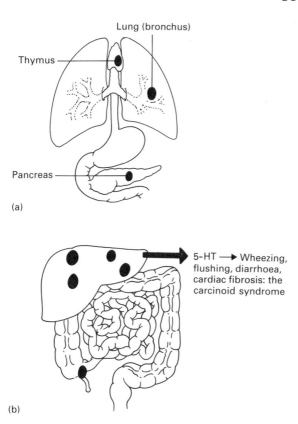

Fig. 6.1. Carcinoid tumours and the carcinoid syndrome. (a) Carcinoid tumours in derivatives of the embryological foregut secrete peptide hormones, such as ACTH. Small cell anaplastic (oat cell) carcinoma of the bronchus is a malignant form of carcinoid tumour. (b) Carcinoid tumours of the hindgut (small bowel and appendix) secrete amines (5-HT). If there are liver metastases, the 5-HT enters the systemic circulation and causes the carcinoid syndrome.

carcinoid tumours of the small bowel present with the effects of excessive secretion of vasoactive substances: the carcinoid syndrome (Fig. 6.1).

The carcinoid syndrome

The tumours which cause the carcinoid syndrome are derived from the argentaffin (silver-staining) cells of the bowel, and these are commonest in the appendix. Small tumours (< 1 cm diameter) are usually benign and are often found incidentally at appendicectomy. Larger ones (especially when > 3 cm) may metastasize.

Clinical

The symptoms of the carcinoid syndrome occur only when the excessive 5-HT and kinins reach the systemic (as opposed to the portal) circulation, and this nearly always means it occurs only when there are extensive liver metastases. It is not known which of the various vasoactive substances produced by the tumours is responsible for the symptoms. The symptoms are the result, however, of widespread changes in smooth-muscle contractility — cutaneous flushing, sweating, hypotension and dizziness, bronchospasm, and gastrointestinal spasm resulting in colic and diarrhoea. These symptoms are typically paroxysmal, with attacks being precipitated by exercise or emotion but also by the ingestion of certain foods, such as cheese. In chronic cases endocardial fibrosis occurs, affecting the right side of the heart and leading to pulmonary stenosis and right-heart failure.

Diagnosis

The clinical diagnosis is confirmed by the finding of excessive urinary excretion of 5-hydroxyindoleacetic acid (5HIAA). The sample for 5HIAA measurement requires acid as a preservative.

Treatment

The only effective treatment is tumour removal. Tumours causing the carcinoid syndrome tend to be slow-growing, and slow-growing tumours are typically resistant to both radiotherapy and chemotherapy. Many drugs have been tried to control the symptoms, including phenothiazines and other antihistamines, histamine receptor blockers and sympathetic blockers, but without spectacular success. Similarly, the use of agents which reduce 5-HT synthesis, such as parachlorophenylalanine and methyldopa, does not produce invariable improvement. Symptomatic improvement may follow arterial embolization of hepatic metastases.

FLUSHING ATTACKS

People often complain of flushing or sweating attacks, and most have no serious medical problem. It can be difficult to be sure how many tests should be done in order to exclude rare and unlikely conditions.

Anxiety

People who are anxious and tense may complain of hot, dizzy attacks. Some may be associated with tachycardia or hyperventilation.

Dietary factors

Hot and spicy foods often cause facial sweating, especially in younger people. In some people this can be a cause of great discomfort and distress. The mechanism is unknown.

Menopause

Menopausal flushing is a normal occurrence in 50% of women. The flushes can pre-date the cessation of menstruation and can continue for many months, or years, afterwards. Each flush is associated with a surge in serum gonadotrophin concentrations, but the surge follows the onset of the flush. In other words, the rise in gonadotrophins does not cause the flush — both are probably triggered by the same hypothalamic neurotransmitter.

Unexplained sweating

Some people complain of sweating which remains unexplained. This can occur in the middle of the night and may indicate some autonomic dysfunction, but the mechanism is obscure.

Thyrotoxicosis

Thyrotoxicosis can make people feel hot and sweaty.

Acromegaly

Excessive growth hormone causes increased sebum production: the severity of greasy sweating is a good guide to the activity of the disease.

Hypoglycaemia

Hypoglycaemia may be spontaneous, but is usually induced by hypoglycaemic agents such as insulin and sulphonylurea drugs.

Diabetic autonomic neuropathy

People with diabetes may rarely develop gross sympathetic denervation as part of the syndrome of autonomic neuropathy. They flush when eating (spicy food, or dairy products and cheese), or even just thinking of food. This is called gustatory sweating. It may be associated with other symptoms of sympathetic denervation, such as dizziness on standing (postural hypotension).

Ethanol

Ethanol causes peripheral vasodilatation, as well as increased catecholamine secretion and a tendency to hypoglycaemia.

Other drugs

Any vasodilator drug may cause a feeling of hotness because of peripheral vasodilatation. It is particularly common with calcium-channel blocking drugs such as nifedipine.

Phaeochromocytoma

Paroxysmal release of catecholamines may cause sweating, in association with pallor, trembling, anxiety and raised blood pressure.

Carcinoid syndrome

Paroxysmal release of 5-HT and other vasoactive amines may cause flushing attacks, together with bronchospasm and diarrhoea.

Chapter 7
The Thymus

The thymus plays a central role in modulating the immune system and in orchestrating the response of the body to injury and to stress. It is itself influenced by the autonomic nervous system, as well as by some circulating hormones: adrenocorticotrophic hormone (ACTH)/cortisol, growth hormone and, possibly, thyroid-stimulating hormone. In turn, the thymus probably plays a key part in modulating the function of some endocrine glands, e.g. the thyroid. This may explain, at least in part, why the size of glands such as the thyroid may increase at times of stress, as well as why autoimmune disease of such glands is so common.

HORMONES OF THE THYMUS

There are a number of related polypeptides in the thymus, referred to collectively as thymosins. Six have been described, but there are probably many more. Details of how they may modify lymphocyte production and the action of other glands, are not known.

DISEASES OF THE THYMUS

Congenital agenesis of the thymus is associated with critical immune deficiency. Tumours of the thymus (thymomas) may be associated with myasthenia gravis, which is an autoimmune disease with antibodies directed at the acetylcholine receptor of muscles motor end-plates. Carcinoid tumours occur in the thymus, and can secrete peptide hormones such as ACTH and cause ectopic humoral syndromes.

Chapter 8
Diabetes Mellitus

Diabetes is a disease which affects the metabolism of carbohydrate, protein and fat, and which can cause complications in every tissue and organ of the body. It is a disease of insulin deficiency (total or relative), and it is diagnosed by demonstrating a high blood sugar level (hyperglycaemia). The history of diabetes is detailed in Table 8.1.

DIAGNOSIS

Although diabetes is a complex metabolic disorder, diagnosis rests entirely on blood glucose.

Casual blood glucose concentration

In people with symptoms, it is sufficient to demonstrate > 11 mmol litre^{-1} in a casual venous sample. If there are no symptoms, two elevated results must be obtained.

Fasting blood glucose

A fasting blood sugar is elevated if it is > 7.0 mmol litre^{-1}.

Table 8.1. History of diabetes

1500 BC	Date of Ebers papyrus. The papyrus describes abnormal polyuria, and was bought by Ebers in Luxor in the 1870s.
500 BC	Diabetes described ('honey urine') in the *Ayur Veda* of Susruta. Also recognized by the Chinese.
AD 50	Celsus described abnormal polyuria
60	Clear description by Aretaeus of Cappadocia
1000	Avicenna noted the association between diabetes, skin infections and impotence.
1682	Brunner observed polydipsia and polyuria in a pancreatectomized dog
1788	Cawley suggested the pancreas may be involved
1869	Islets described by Langerhans
1889	Minkowski and von Mering noted that pancreatectomy caused diabetes in the dog
1909	de Meyer called the postulated pancreatic factor 'insulin'
1921	Paulesco extracted insulin. Banting and Best extracted insulin, purified it and used it to treat diabetes in a dog

Glucose tolerance test

If casual or fasting samples are equivocal, blood glucose is measured after an oral glucose load (75 g glucose — 380 ml Lucozade — on an empty stomach). If blood glucose is 11 mmol litre^{-1} at 2 hours the person has diabetes. If it is less than 7.0 mmol litre^{-1} (in capillary blood), the person is normal. If it is between 7.0 and 11 mmol litre^{-1}, the person has 'impaired glucose tolerance'.

Impaired glucose tolerance

Impaired glucose tolerance (IGT) is associated with an increased risk of macrovascular (atherosclerotic) disease, but not with other complications of diabetes. Approximately 10% of people with IGT convert to diabetes each year. People with IGT should be advised to lose weight if necessary, eat healthily, take regular exercise and not smoke. They should be kept under surveillance.

Presentation of diabetes

Clinical

The symptoms of hyperglycaemia are listed in Table 8.2. Dizziness in the elderly is an important symptom, as is an increase in night cramps. Change in visual acuity is caused by change in the glucose content of the lens, cornea and vitreous, with altered refraction. It settles over 2–3 months when normoglycaemia is achieved.

Pruritis vulvae may indicate vaginal candidiasis, but it can result from hyperglycaemia alone — especially in older women. Superficial dysuria can also occur in women without there being any infection. Candida is extremely rare in men, unless they have diabetes. Hyperglycaemia should be excluded in any man with balanitis or late-onset phimosis.

TYPES OF DIABETES

There are a number of different types of diabetes (Table 8.3). They have different causes, and different clinical features.

Table 8.2. Symptoms of hyperglycaemia

Polyuria, nocturia
Symptoms of salt and water depletion
  Thirst
  Dizziness (in the elderly)
  Cramps (especially at night)
Tiredness
Altered visual acuity
Symptoms of infection
  Pruritis vulvae
  Balanitis
  Boils
  Infection of skin and nails

Table 8.3. Types of diabetes

Type I	Insulin-dependent, ketosis-prone
Type II	Non-insulin dependent
Gestational	Diabetes present in pregnancy which remits after delivery
Secondary	Secondary to conditions causing insulin resistance (e.g. acromegaly, Cushing's syndrome)
Other disease of the pancreas	Diabetes caused by pancreatectomy or pancreatitis, haemochromatosis
Other congenital or inherited syndromes	e.g. Prader–Willi, DIDMOAD and Lawrence–Moon–Biedl syndromes; Friedreich's ataxia, dystrophia myotonica
Target organ resistance	Receptor and post-receptor defects

Type I diabetes

People with Type I diabetes have total or near-total loss of pancreatic insulin.

Prevalence

People with Type I diabetes tend to be young, but can be any age from infancy to senescence. About 1 child in 800 has diabetes, boys being slightly more affected than girls. It is becoming more common. There are peaks of new cases each year in the spring and the autumn.

Clinical

Sufferers tend to be young, and the onset is relatively quick. They may have had symptoms for only a few days. Because they are insulin-deficient, they metabolize fat to provide energy; they thus lose weight and are thin. They also have ketones in the urine. If ketones accumulate excessively, they develop ketoacidosis.

Ketoacidosis

The patient with ketoacidosis is dangerously ill and will die unless treated with urgency. They are dehydrated (from the diuretic effect of hyperglycaemia), and acidotic: Kussmaul respiration, with the smell of ketones on their breath. They will feel sick, and may vomit.

Non-specific abdominal pain (with elevation in serum amylase and neutrophil leucocytosis) occurs in ketoacidosis. The patient may be drowsy, confused or comatose. There may be signs of an intercurrent illness (e.g. chest infection) which has precipitated the crisis.

Causes of Type I diabetes

Inheritance

There is a genetic factor which predisposes an individual, but the inheritance is not strong. In 80% of cases there is no one else in the family with the disease. If a diabetic woman has a baby, the risk of the child developing Type I diabetes is 1–2% (8–10 times normal). The children of men with Type I diabetes have a 5% risk (reason unknown). The siblings of affected children have about a 1 in 10 chance of developing the disease as well. The identical twin of a diabetic has a 50% chance.

Type I diabetes is associated with a number of HLA types, and their significance varies with different populations: DR3 and DR4 are most prominent in Caucasians.

Autoimmunity

The inherited factor in Type I diabetes is thought to be a predisposition to autoimmune destruction of the islets. The process involves both T-cells (cell-mediated) and B-cells (humoral). Islet cell antibodies (ICA) may be found in the serum of Type I diabetics at about the time of diagnosis, but they become undetectable later. The pancreas of a new Type I diabetic has extensive lymphocytic infiltration: the islets are destroyed.

Environmental

As in all autoimmune disease, it is thought that an environmental trigger (or triggers) is necessary for activation of the process. Virus infections have been implicated but no single virus has been found responsible.

Type II diabetes

In Type II diabetes there is a relative lack of insulin. The insulin which is present is sufficient to prevent excessive fat metabolism, and the person is not at risk of ketosis.

It is not clear how often total insulin secretion is reduced in Type II diabetes, and how often insulin secretion is relatively normal but insufficient because of peripheral antagonism to its action. Measured insulin concentrations are usually higher than normal, but this may be because of cross-reaction with insulin-related peptides.

Prevalence

Type II diabetes is more common than Type I. It is also more common with advancing age, affecting up to 20% in their 80s. Type II is particularly prevalent in people who are of Indian origin — affecting up to 20% at the age of 60.

Clinical

People with Type II diabetes tend to be older and fatter. They may have lost a little weight before presentation (up to 4 kg), but not much. They may have had symptoms for several weeks or months before diagnosis. Alternatively, they may be symptom-free and only detected on routine screening. It is estimated that there is one undiagnosed case for every diagnosed one in the community.

Because the disease may be occult for long periods before detection, complications (retinopathy, foot ulceration, proteinuria) may be present at the time of diagnosis. Because of their age and tendency to obesity, people with Type II diabetes are especially prone to macrovascular complications.

Causes of Type II diabetes

Inheritance

Inheritance plays a greater part in Type II diabetes. Affected people are much more likely to have an affected family member. The inheritance pattern is not clear, and there is no link with any particular HLA type.

Autoimmunity

Autoimmunity is not a feature of Type II diabetes. ICA are negative and there is no lymphocytic infiltration of the pancreas. Histologically the islets may be normal, or may show perivascular infiltration with amyloid (50%). This amyloid is composed mainly of islet amyloid polypeptide (IAPP, amylin) which is a 37-amino acid peptide which is normally co-secreted with insulin from the islets of Langerhans. The significance of the amyloid, and of IAPP, is unknown.

Environmental

Environmental factors will precipitate diabetes in those predisposed to it. The most important environmental factors are diet (high carbohydrate) and obesity. Thiazide diuretics and β-blockers (which are prescribed liberally in the elderly) may also precipitate the disease because they impair insulin secretion.

Maturity-onset diabetes of young people

Some young people have non-insulin dependent diabetes. This is called maturity-onset diabetes of young people (MODY). It appears to be inherited as an autosomal dominant with incomplete penetrance. Such people seem to be relatively protected from complications.

Gestational diabetes

Some women develop diabetes in pregnancy, but it clears as soon as the baby is born. This is called gestational diabetes. The neonates tend to be large (macrosomia) but relatively immature at birth. There is an increased risk of fetal loss and of maternal morbidity, but this is reduced by aggressive control of blood glucose during pregnancy.

Some women have macrosomic babies (> 9 lb, 4.5 kg) without having had any evidence of gestational diabetes. A woman who has such a heavy baby is more likely to develop diabetes in later life but the relative risk is not known. On the other hand, 35% of women presenting with Type II diabetes in later life will have had macrosomic infants years earlier.

Diabetes and other diseases of the pancreas

Chronic pancreatitis (which may be painless) may be diagnosed by the appearance of pancreatic calcification on abdominal X-ray. Acute pancreatitis can cause diabetes (just as diabetes, with hypertriglyceridaemia, is one of the causes of acute pancreatitis). Diabetes will occur following resection of the pancreas.

Haemochromatosis is a congenital disorder of iron transport characterized by the deposition of iron in many tissues, including the pancreas. Because of the associated brownish pigmentation of the skin, the condition was once called 'bronze diabetes'. Glucagonomas and somatostatinomas are also associated with diabetes.

Type II diabetes may be a presenting symptom of carcinoma of the pancreas. The reason is not clear, because it does not require the whole gland to be replaced by tumour. Carcinoma of the pancreas is not more common in people with established diabetes.

ASSESSMENT OF THE NEWLY DIAGNOSED DIABETIC

Diabetes is usually suspected because glucose is detected in the urine (glycosuria). The first task is to prove the diagnosis by demonstrating hyperglycaemia. The second is to make sure that the person does not have ketonuria.

Blood glucose can be estimated using a stick test, but a sample should be sent to the laboratory for confirmation. The height of the blood sugar is no guide to the severity of the condition. Someone with diet-controllable Type II diabetes may well have a blood glucose of 25 mmol litre^{-1} at presentation. The need for urgency is indicated by two things:

1   The person's general health: are they obviously ill?
2   The presence of ketonuria.

When a person is found to have glycosuria, they should have their urine checked immediately for ketones. If the result is + + or + + + , an urgent referral should be made by telephone to a specialist. In Type I diabetes it is usual to start treatment with insulin the same day. If the person has no markers of insulin dependence (Table 8.4), the condition can be managed with less urgency, and the priorities of management can be determined (see p. 150).

Table 8.4. Features of Types I and II diabetes

Features suggesting that diabetes is Type I (insulin-dependent)
Ketonuria with/without ketoacidosis
Thinness
Weight loss
Short history of symptoms
Young age
Positive ICA

Features suggesting that diabetes is Type II (non-insulin-dependent)
Ketones negative or only trace positive
Fatness
Weight loss minimal (< 4 kg)
Longer history
Previous gestational diabetes or macrosomia
Stronger family history
Negative or weak positive ICA

MANAGEMENT

Management of hyperglycaemic emergencies

There are three different types of hyperglycaemic emergency:

1 Ketoacidosis (DKA).
2 Hyperosmolar non-ketotic (HONK) coma.
3 Lactic acidosis.

In all three the patient is obviously ill. The mortality is high in all three conditions, and urgent referral to a specialist centre is mandatory.

Ketoacidosis

The principles of treatment are:

1 Rehydration with saline until glucose falls.
2 Insulin administration
   (a) to inhibit lipolysis and ketogenesis
   (b) to lower blood glucose.
3 Administration of K^+, after the initial stage.
4 Continued administration of glucose and insulin until the ketones are cleared and the patient is eating normally.
5 Treatment of any precipitating cause.

A standard regimen for the treatment of ketoacidosis is given in Table 8.5. The guidelines will need to be modified according to the patient's age and health. Blood sugar and potassium need checking hourly initially.

Table 8.5. Treatment of ketoacidosis

---

i.v. normal saline: 5 litres in approx. 15 hours
1 litre in 30 minutes
1 litre in 60 minutes
1 litre in 2 hours
1 litre in 4 hours
1 litre in 8 hours

i.v. soluble insulin:
50 U in 50 ml saline — syringe pump
6 U hour^{-1} until blood glucose < 12 mmol litre^{-1}
3 U hour^{-1} adjusted on the basis of response
Insulin requirements will fall as ketones clear — eventually to 1–2 U hour^{-1}

i.v. potassium:
Although plasma potassium concentration may be high at presentation it will fall as insulin is given. Total body potassium is low.
   Withhold potassium until plasma K^+ < 5.5 mmol litre^{-1}
   Give 20 mmol KCl hour^{-1} or more:
   enough to keep plasma potassium > 4.0 and < 5.5 mmol litre^{-1}
Nasogastric tube (if consciousness clouded)
Antibiotics if indicated
ECG monitor

The hardest part of management is on the 2nd–3rd days. If the person is transferred back to s.c. insulin too soon, ketosis will recur.

Hyperosmolar coma

Hyperosmolar non-ketotic coma is uncommon. The patient is usually previously undiagnosed, and although blood sugar is initially very high (50–80 mmol litre^{-1}), is usually non-insulin-dependent. The cause is not known. It rarely recurs.

Heparin should be given s.c. to prevent venous thrombosis (unless there is proliferative retinopathy).

Treat with i.v. half-strength saline, and i.v. insulin infusion. The patient will usually be able to come off insulin before leaving hospital.

Lactic acidosis

Lactic acidosis is extremely rare. The patient is acidotic because of excessive lactate accumulation. This happens only if their illness is associated with extensive tissue anoxia (critical disease of heart, lung or kidney). It may be more likely if people with renal failure are given metformin, but this is unproven.

The patient will be acidotic but without ketones. They will be extremely ill, and mortality is > 50%. Treat with infusion of isotonic $NaHCO_3$ and i.v. insulin.

Management of the new Type I who is relatively well

A newly diagnosed insulin-dependent diabetic with ketosis (i.e. ketones in the urine), but without ketoacidosis (i.e. clinically well; normal blood pH) should be referred for urgent specialist care, but does not need to be admitted to hospital — it is better if they are not.

They should be taught to give their first insulin injection themselves. Once the injection is given they will have conquered much of their terror and will be able to listen to what is being said.

Management on day 1

Much of what is said and done depends on the individual, but it is a mistake to say or do too much too quickly.

1   Teach patient to inject themselves with a small dose of insulin.

2   8–10 U s.c. (less in slight children) twice daily of soluble or isophane insulin will restore well-being and abolish the risk of progression to ketoacidosis. There is a chance of hypoglycaemia, but it is a small one.

3   Advise them to eat regularly, but to avoid sweet things.

4   Advise them not to drive for a few days — unless they are quite confident and the risk of hypoglycaemia is negligible.

5   Warn about the small chance of hypoglycaemia, and tell them to carry sweets or dextrose tablets in case it occurs.

6   Advise them to inform the DVLA and their insurance company if they are continuing to drive.

7   Give them your phone number and/or other contact.

8   Phone their GP and tell them what has been done.

9   Arrange follow-up.

Note that no attempt is made to achieve normoglycaemia, or to teach the patient how to measure anything — it is not necessary at this stage. The initial priority is to prevent ketoacidosis and restore well-being.

Management during the next few weeks

1 More is taught on the nature of diabetes, its causes and its problems.

2 More is taught about food adjustment and the effects of exercise on blood sugar.

3 The patient is taught about the concept of a normal blood sugar, and how to try and maintain it.

4 They are taught how to measure blood and urine for sugar — to show that they have achieved normoglycaemia.

5 The reason for maintaining normal blood sugar is explained: it is not enough to abolish symptoms, the aim is also to prevent complications.

6 The need is stressed to bend diabetes to accomodate a relatively normal lifestyle.

7 Question-answering, reassurance.

The eventual aim is to enable the person to achieve a normal blood sugar for as much of the time as possible, to feel well, and to adjust to their illness. To be done well, this usually requires the services of an expert multidisciplinary team (doctor, nurse, dietitian, chiropodist and others).

An expert team will pace the educational process to the requirements of the individual, often using a checklist to make sure that they have covered all topics. An expert team will also expect the usual sequence of reactions experienced by newly treated diabetics (Table 8.6).

In the end, each diabetic will decide for themselves how much they are going to allow the disease to control their lives. Having been taught, they will make a percentage decision on the value or otherwise of striving for close control.

Parents of diabetic children are especially vulnerable. Mothers in particular may feel ineradicable guilt for (a) passing on the diabetes gene, and (b) having done something wrong in the child's upbringing. They are continually frightened lest their other children develop the disease. They may be especially frustrated by the impossibility of achieving good glucose control (and it is impossible in children because of their explosive lifestyle), and fear that they are therefore predisposing the child to complications in later life. Parents need as much support and encouragement as diabetic children do.

Table 8.6. Sequence of emotional reactions which may be experienced by newly treated insulin-dependent diabetics

---

Early
Horror
Pride at self-injection
Pleasure from improved health

Later
Anger: Why me?
Anger at having to cope with the injections, food, monitoring
Fear of a lifetime with diabetes
Fear of complications
Annoyance: at the ignorance of ordinary people; about loaded insurance premiums, etc.

Management of the new type II diabetic

The new Type II diabetic is not dangerously ill, and there is usually no need for urgent referral to a specialist centre. The aims of management are given below. The speed with which they are covered depends on the patient, their needs and the resources available.

1 Explain the diagnosis and its significance.

2 Emphasize that it can be controlled, but that it will not go away. There is no such thing as 'mild diabetes'.

3 Treat symptoms (if any):

    (a) Symptoms of hyperglycaemia can be controlled with diet and/or tablets.

    (b) Symptomatic treatment, e.g. for candidiasis.

4 Teach about the aims of management and monitoring (urine testing is usually sufficient for Type II diabetes).

5 Cover as much as is appropriate of the education checklist.

6 Answer questions. Reassure — especially about complications (about which people sometimes acquire wrong information).

7 Arrange follow-up.

Management of gestational diabetes

Gestational diabetes is treated intensively. All affected women should see diabetes specialist staff together with obstetric staff in joint clinics. The object of treatment is to achieve normoglycaemia, and the blood sugar is likely to be highest 1–2 hours after each meal. The woman is advised to avoid sweet foods, and thus reduce the post-prandial rise in blood glucose. She is taught to measure her blood sugar 6–7 times daily, twice a week. If diet does not reduce the post-prandial peak, she should be treated with short-acting soluble insulin given s.c. before meals. Longer-acting isophane is given before bed if the glucose is high (> 8 mmol litre^{-1}) before breakfast.

The urine should be checked for ketones at each clinic visit. Occasionally, women who develop hyperglycaemia in pregnancy have coincidental Type I diabetes.

Management of diabetes in ethnic minorities

The principles of management are no different from those of management of Caucasians. However, problems arise from difficulty in communication, and from lack of insight by professionals into social and cultural differences between them and their patients.

There is no language barrier with Afro-Caribbeans, but there may be significant differences in attitude to life, and in health-care priorities between them and the average Caucasian professional. Blacks are often accused of non-compliance, when the main failing might be that of the professional who suggests inappropriate treatment.

There are often major problems of communication with people who are ethnically Indian — especially with Muslim women who are first-generation immigrants. Moreover, many Indians and Pakistani immigrants come from relatively rural, disadvantaged areas.

It is essential for the health-care team to understand something of the religious and cultural factors which may temper the ability of the Asian patient to manage his or her diabetes well. Some of these are simple: failure to attend the clinic because older Muslim women will not leave the house during the day, because the clinic is held on a Friday, or because they have gone back to Pakistan for a prolonged holiday. Some are more complex: the concepts of 'hot' conditions and 'cold' conditions, and the appropriateness of different foods and treatments in their management.

The failure of doctors to appreciate differences in social and cultural values is not, of course, limited to their dealings with people of different race. Doctors, and especially hospital doctors, may sometimes have precious little insight into the realities of life for many British-born Caucasians!

DIETARY MODIFICATION IN DIABETES

The word 'diet' is regarded by people as a sort of punishment: something which they do not find easy but which other people expect them to do. They feel guilty (or aggressive and defensive) when they fail. The world 'diet' must be used carefully. It is better to talk about 'food' and 'eating'.

Objectives

The objectives are fourfold:
1 Reduced intake of readily assimilable sugars (to reduce post-prandial peaks).
2 Eating regularly to avoid hypoglycaemia if on insulin or tablets.
3 Weight reduction in the overweight.
4 'Healthy eating': high-fibre, low in saturated fats, moderate alcohol, etc.
Such simple advice can be given by any health-care professional, but all insulin-dependent and many non-insulin-dependent diabetics should be given the opportunity of discussing their eating habits with a dietitian.

Effectiveness of dietary advice

Only 20% of people lose weight when advised, and two-thirds of these will have regained their original weight after 2 years (restoration of 'le milieu postérieur' — to parody Claude Bernard). As long as professionals recognize that this is usual, they will be less frustrated or angered by the failure of any individual to get their weight down. It is interesting that blood glucose may well fall in response to diet, even though overall weight does not. This may reflect increased sensitivity to insulin from the reduced carbohydrate content of the diet.

TABLET TREATMENT OF DIABETES: ORAL HYPOGLYCAEMIC AGENTS

Tablets are only suitable for Type II diabetes. They should not be used in gestational diabetes, and do not work in Type I. Oral insulin is not available, although attempts have been made to give it nasally.

Sulphonylureas

Sulphonylurea drugs lower blood glucose by stimulating pancreatic insulin release. If the pancreas has no insulin (as in Type I diabetes), they will not work.

There are a large number of different preparations (see Table 8.7), but most doctors will use only one or two. Chlorpropamide and glibenclamide are long-acting and need be given only once a day, which is an advantage. However, long-acting drugs are much more likely to cause hypoglycaemia. Such hypoglycaemia may be clinically obvious (see Table 6.4), but equally may not: the elderly may complain of dizziness, confusion, headache, or may even present with symptoms and signs of a transient ischaemic attack (TIA).

Such problems are less likely with shorter-acting preparations such as tolbutamide or gliclazide. Gliclazide is probably the treatment of choice in renal failure, because it is cleared in the bile. The problem with tolbutamide is that the tablet is a large one. The problem with gliclazide is that it is more expensive.

All sulphonylureas cause weight gain, but the problem is worse with glibenclamide and chlorpropamide.

Metformin

Metformin is a biguanide and acts by increasing peripheral uptake of glucose while reducing hepatic glucose output. It does not increase insulin secretion by the pancreas — it makes it work better. It can be used on its own or as an adjunct to sulphonylureas. Metformin has to be taken in two or three doses through the day. The tablets are large and may cause nausea or gastrointestinal upset. It has less of a tendency to cause weight gain than sulphonylureas (perhaps because it puts people off their food!), and is indicated in the obese Type II diabetic who fails to achieve normoglycaemia by diet alone.

There is a theoretical risk of metformin precipitating lactic acidosis, and hence it is not given to people at risk of acidosis or tissue anoxia (severe cardiorespiratory disease, liver disease, renal failure).

Table 8.7. Some sulphonylurea preparations

Short-acting
Short-acting preparations have to be taken two or three times daily. They may reduce the post-prandial peak of blood glucose better than long-acting ones. They may also have less of an effect on weight gain.

Tablet	Dose range (mg)
Tolbutamide	500–1500
Gliclazide	40–320

Gliclazide is excreted in bile, and can be used in renal failure.

Long-acting
Long-acting preparations need to be taken only once each day. There is an increased risk of hypoglycaemia if a meal is missed. They may also have more of an effect on weight gain than shorter-acting preparations.

Tablet	Dose range (mg)
Chlorpropamide	100–500
Glibenclamide	2.5–15

Choice of oral hypoglycaemic agent
There are four sorts of people with non-insulin-dependent diabetes.

Overweight person without symptoms
Diet is the first-line treatment. Post-prandial peaks will be lowered by reduced intake of sweet food, and insulin resistance will be lessened as they lose weight.

Overweight person with symptoms
Although many doctors advise an initial trial of diet alone, symptoms will resolve more quickly if the patient is given tablets. Metformin (500 mg b.d.–850 mg t.d.s.) is preferable to sulphonylureas because it is less likely to worsen obesity. An attempt should be made to withdraw the tablets after 2–3 weeks.

Thin person without symptoms
The main object of management is to achieve normal blood sugar (as well as to watch for ketonuria or other signs of insulin dependence). Diet alone may be sufficient, but they may need a sulphonylurea (e.g. tolbutamide 250 mg b.d.–500 mg t.d.s.; glibenclamide 2.5 mg daily–15 mg daily; gliclazide 40 mg b.d.–160 mg b.d.; or chlorpropamide 100 mg daily–500 mg daily).

Thin person with symptoms
These people need treatment with sulphonylureas with or without metformin. Some later need insulin.

INSULIN TREATMENT
If insulin is given simply to control symptoms, it may given once daily. If it is given in an attempt to achieve normoglycaemia, it needs to be given two, three or four times daily. There have been vogues for continuous administration via s.c or i.v. cannulae, but these have never been popular in the UK.

Types of insulin
The types of insulin available are shown in Table 8.8.

Species of insulin
Most insulin used in the UK is structurally identical to human insulin, but is produced by genetic engineering of bacteria or yeasts. Porcine insulin is extracted from pigs. Extracted beef insulin is still available, and is the main type of insulin used in non-industrialized countries. Engineered human and porcine insulins have the advantage of being pure, less dependent on animal exploitation, and ultimately cheaper. (Table 8.9).

Choice of insulin regimen
The choice is usually left to specialists. It is usual to start the treatment of Type I diabetes with two injections a day, before breakfast and before the evening meal, of 8–10 U s.c. of soluble or isophane.

If post-prandial hyperglycaemia is a problem, then either the amount of food in the meal should be reduced or the amount of soluble insulin given before the meal

Table 8.8. Types of insulin

Soluble
Short-acting, clear, neutral
Duration of action 0.5–8 hours
   (sometimes longer)

Actrapid
Velosulin
Humulin S
Hypurin neutral

Isophane
Medium-acting, cloudy
Duration of action 2–15 hours
   (sometimes longer)

Protaphane
Insulatard
Humulin I
Hypurin isophane

Lente
Longer-acting, cloudy
Duration of action 6–24 hours
   (sometimes longer)

Monotard
Humulin Zn
Hypurin lente

Crystalline
Very long acting
Duration of action 24–36 hours

Ultratard

Fixed mixtures
Manufacturers of the above preparations
market mixtures of soluble and isophane:
Actrapid and Protaphane
Velosulin and Insulatard
Humulin series

Actraphane, Penmix series
Mixtard
M1, M2, M3, M4

Others
There are a number of other preparations
but none are widely used

Table 8.9. Sources of insulin

Human	Porcine	Beef
Actrapid	Velosulin	Hypurin preps
Humulin preps	Insulatard	
Protaphane	Mixtard	
Monotard		

Velosulin, Insulatard and Mixtard are also available as human forms

is increased. If the blood glucose is high before the evening meal or first thing in the morning, then the dose of isophane (or lente, if used) needs to be increased. It is a simple matter to devise an insulin regimen for people, using one, two or three injections a day. (Fig. 8.1). Doses are adjusted according to their requirements (more with more food, less if they are taking more exercise), and to the response of the blood sugar.

Blood sugar profile

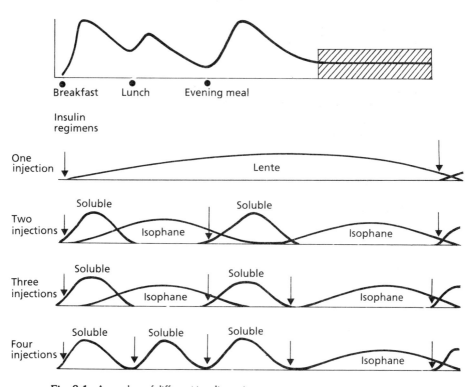

Fig. 8.1. A number of different insulin regimens.

In general, once-daily injections will prevent ketoacidosis and will control symptoms in many, but are not flexible enough to achieve close glycaemic control. Injections four times a day (usually using a pen injector) are inconvenient but are preferred by most young people nevertheless. It is easier for them to live a variable lifestyle and yet still keep their blood sugars normal: it is easier to bend diabetes to fit their life, rather than bend their lives to fit diabetes.

Pen injectors

Pen injectors are gadgets for the easy transport and injection of insulin — especially appropriate for people who frequently have to have injections away from home. They have been enormously successful and have made it much easier for people to adapt to multiple-injection regimens.

Hypoglycaemia

If a person on tablets or insulin alters his or her habits in any way, there is a risk that the blood glucose will fall too low and he or she will go hypoglycaemic. Hypoglycaemia may thus be precipitated by extra exercise, missing meals, or alcohol.

If the person drinks alcohol to excess one evening, they will develop hyperglycaemia while drinking (because of the increased carbohydrate intake), but will go hypoglycaemic during the night because alcohol inhibits the ability of the body to maintain blood glucose by gluconeogenesis. Sometimes the hypoglycaemic attack occurs during the next morning.

Symptoms

The symptoms of hypoglycaemia are given in Table 6.4, although attention is drawn to different presentations in the elderly.

Treatment

Hypoglycaemia is treated by consuming any sweet food or drink. If it is not possible for the person to recognize the attack and have some food, it may be necessary for others to try and give them sips of sweet drinks (they can be absorbed from the mouth, and recovery can follow quickly after giving only tiny amounts). Parenteral treatment with glucagon 1 mg (s.c. or i.m.) may be necessary, or even intravenous glucose.

If untreated, hypoglycaemia will recover spontaneously from increased glycogenolysis and gluconeogenesis induced by catecholamines, growth hormone and cortisol.

Prevention

If hypoglycaemic attacks occur regularly, then the diet or insulin dose should be modified, or tablets should be stopped altogether.

Significance

Hypoglycaemic attacks ('hypos' or 'reactions') are the most feared complication of all for people taking insulin. If they have a bad hypo and lose consciousness, they may have a fit and be incontinent. They lose independence and self-esteem. They are embarrassed to expose a 'weakness' to family, friends or people at work. They lose half a day in a hospital casualty department. They may lose their driving licence or their job. They may have an accident and do themselves, or someone else, an injury.

It follows that fear of hypoglycaemia is a much more potent determinant of behaviour in an insulin-treated diabetic than fear of possible long-term complications. It is one of the main reasons why many young people give up striving for close control, feel happier with a rather higher blood glucose, and tend to adjust treatment simply on how they feel. It is natural behaviour — even though it may worsen the long-term prognosis.

Hypoglycaemia unawareness

Some people taking insulin lose their warning symptoms of hypoglycaemia. They are not then able to recognize the onset of a hypoglycaemic attack, and this can be extremely dangerous. If a person loses warning symptoms, they should not drive. The cause of the loss of warning is not known. It has been suggested that it may accompany a change of insulin species from porcine or bovine to human types, but this is not proven. In some cases it is the result of autonomic neuropathy, but such cases are very rare.

It is possible that in some cases it is the result of close glycaemic control: the lower a person has managed to keep their average blood sugar, the less it has to fall before it goes too low, and the less likely it is that warning symptoms will be triggered in time. Never was effort more poisonously rewarded.

If people have lost warning symptoms, they should strive for less close control and should be encouraged to measure their own blood sugar more often.

COMPLICATIONS OF DIABETES

There are three broad types of complication: psychosocial, problems of blood glucose control, and chronic complications.

Psychosocial

The main problem for young people is the knowledge that they have a disease when there is great pressure to be both healthy and the same as everyone else. In some cases the consciousness of being 'abnormal' produces a sense of isolation.

There is a persistent frustration felt as a result of the disease, and also with doctors and nurses. Professionals — who do not have diabetes themselves — exhort you to lead a normal life and at the same time to try and control your blood sugar closely. However, you know that if you control your blood sugar tightly, there is the ever-present worry of hypoglycaemia, and also that it is impossible to lead a normal life with diabetes.

The problem for older people is different and usually centres on having complications, or the fear of them.

Problems of blood-sugar control

1 Ketoacidosis (see p. 127).
2 Hyperosmolar coma (HONK) (see p. 128).
3 Lactic acidosis (see p. 128).
4 Hypoglycaemia (see p. 135).
5 Chronic inability to control hyperglycaemia — in both Type I and Type II diabetes.

Chronic inability to control blood sugar

Some people find it impossible to control their blood sugar satisfactorily. In the case of Type II diabetes (usually obese), the blood sugar is persistently high despite maximum oral therapy (or even insulin). Failure to adhere to dietary restriction is a factor, and so is insulin resistance.

In Type I diabetes, blood sugar may swing from hyperglycaemia to hypoglycaemia, despite the person's best attempts to stabilize it. Such people are sometimes best advised to stop trying for close control, and to concentrate on being symptom-free.

Brittle diabetes

'Brittle diabetes' is the term sometimes given to people who have recurrent major swings in blood sugar, and who require frequent admission to hospital with either ketoacidosis or hypoglycaemia.

Brittle diabetes is most often seen in adolescents and young people, and often proves transient, leading many to conclude that either subconscious or manipulative behaviour is a factor. It may be a 'cry for help'. The person should be offered opportunities to talk, but confrontation is not likely to be beneficial. Attempts at family therapy may open a can of worms.

Chronic complications of diabetes

The changes of diabetes affect every tissue and every organ. These can produce clinically significant complications. In people with Type I diabetes, it is unusual for them to occur in the first 5 years. In Type II diabetes — which may have been occult for a number of years — complications may be present at diagnosis. The main chronic complications are listed in Table 8.10.

Pathogenesis

Several processes contribute to the development of complications.

Ischaemia

Diabetes is associated with abnormal capillary function. Hyperglycaemia allows the increased transudation of albumin across capillary walls. In the longer term capillaries develop thickening of the basement membrane, and this impairs the transfer of nutrients to the tissues. This basement membrane thickening makes the capillary inflexible and less distensible, and thrombosis occurs. The tendency to tissue ischaemia is worsened by the association of this 'microvascular disease' with increased atherogenesis ('macrovascular disease').

Glycosylation

The non-enzymatic attachment of carbohydrate to protein is increased in chronic hyperglycaemia. Glycosylation of collagen causes widespread changes in tissue elasticity. Glycosylation of other proteins, including those in the basement membrane and cellular enzymes, must also be important.

Metabolic

The accumulation of carbohydrate in cells results in increased formation of sorbitol via the enzyme aldose reductase (see Fig. 8.2). The accumulation of sorbitol is toxic to cells, especially neurons.

Brain

Widespread capillary dysfunction renders the brain more susceptible to ischaemic or hypoglycaemic damage. Stroke is twice as common. Mortality from stroke is double.

Heart

Ischaemic heart disease

There is an increased tendency to atherogenesis in diabetes. The risk of myocardial infarction is twofold for men and fourfold for women. Diabetics who are

Table 8.10. Chronic complications of diabetes

Brain	Microvascular disease causing cortical ischaemia Stroke
Heart	Ischaemic heart disease Diabetic cardiomyopathy
Blood pressure	Hypertension probably more common
Peripheral vessels	Claudication Gangrene
Renal tract	Renal failure Papillary necrosis Recurrent infection
Gonad	Possible hormonal changes
Penis	Impotence
Liver	Fatty infiltration Abnormal liver function tests
Skin	Infection Necrobiosis lipoidica Granuloma annulare
Joints	Cheiroarthropathy Frozen shoulder Osteoarthritis
Eye	Cataract Retinopathy

Neuropathies	Somatic
	    Sensory
	    Motor
	    Mononeuropathy
	Autonomic
	Spinal cord

Leucocytes	Neutrophils and monocytes: increased infection
Foot	Ulcers and gangrene

admitted to hospital are twice as likely to die — usually from pulmonary oedema. The increase in pulmonary oedema may reflect associated dysfunction of the myocardium, which is not infarcted. It may also reflect increased transcapillary escape of albumin, which occurs when blood glucose is elevated.

Cardiomyopathy

Specific diffuse cardiomyopathy has been described (leading to left ventricular failure and congestive cardiac failure (CCF)), but its pathological basis is uncertain.

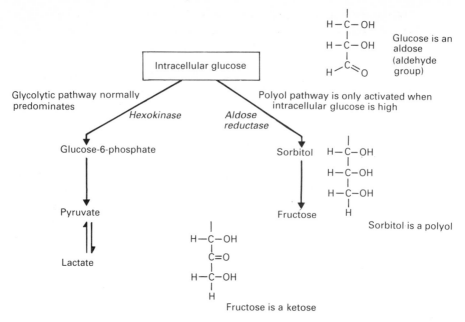

Fig. 8.2. Metabolism of glucose by hexoxinase (glycolysis) or aldose reductase (polyol path).

Blood pressure

Hypertension is more common in newly diagnosed diabetes, and in the elderly. The pathogenesis is complex. Hypertension complicates nephropathy — people with proteinuria have a very greatly increased risk of ischaemic heart disease. Most people with diabetic nephropathy die of vascular disease before they develop critical renal failure.

Peripheral vessels

Diabetics are more likely to develop atherosclerosis leading to distal ischaemia. This may cause claudication, or frank ischaemia of the foot. Atherosclerosis in diabetic legs tends to affect the vessels below the trifurcation of the popliteal. It is harder to treat by bypass surgery and angioplasty.

Renal tract

Glomerulosclerosis and renal failure

Pathology

There is thickening of the glomerular basement membrane, with increased transudation of protein. There is a build-up of extravascular proteinaceous material — thickening of the mesangium. In end-stage renal failure the glomeruli are replaced by amorphous proteinaceous material (glomerulosclerosis; Kimmelstiel–Wilson kidney).

A rise in blood pressure accompanies early nephropathy. As blood pressure rises, the process of nephropathy is accelerated.

Hyperfiltration

In the early years of diabetes there is an increase in glomerular filtration rate (GFR). Those with increased GFR may be those who later develop nephropathy, but it is not proven.

Microalbuminuria

The upper limit of normal albumin excretion is 30 μg min^{-1}. Slight to moderate increases in albumin excretion (30–300 μg min^{-1} — 'microalbuminuria') are undetectable with standard stick tests, but are measurable by immunoassay. Microalbuminuria occurs when the transcapillary escape of albumin is increased as a result of hyperglycaemia. It is also the earliest sign of permanent renal damage. People with microalbuminuria are more likely to develop complications of diabetes than those who do not.

Hypoglycaemia

People with worsening renal failure have a tendency to hypoglycaemic attacks because of reduced renal clearance of insulin. The other endocrinological features of renal disease are summarized on pp. 101–3.

Other complications

People with established nephropathy have a very high prevalence of other complications. They often have proliferative retinopathy and may be blind. They will have peripheral neuropathy, and may have symptomatic autonomic neuropathy. They have a high prevalence of peripheral vascular disease, with foot ulceration.

Treatment

Blood pressure should be treated aggressively. The aim should be to reduce the systolic below 140 mmHg and the diastolic below 85 mmHg. Effective treatment of blood pressure lowers the albumin excretion rate and slows the rate of progression of renal failure. It may also improve the prognosis of cardiovascular disease.

Established renal failure (serum creatinine 600–1000 μmol litre^{-1}) is treated with renal replacement therapy — provided the person's other illnesses are not making their life a misery. Replacement therapy may involve chronic ambulatory peritoneal dialysis (CAPD), haemodialysis or transplantation. The protein content of the diet is reduced, while the carbohydrate is increased.

Gonad

There may be minor abnormalities of gonadal function in both males and females, but they are not marked. In general, women with Type I diabetes will ovulate normally and have a normal conception rate. Men have normal serum testosterone concentrations and sperm count. It is possible, but poorly studied, that women of child-bearing age with Type II (non-insulin-dependent) diabetes, have an increased chance of having polycystic ovary disease (see pp. 210–211).

Impotence

Impotence affects 30–50% of males with diabetes. This is thought to be more common than normal, but it is not known how common impotence is in non-diabetics.

Causes

The causes of impotence are discussed in Chapter 11. It is likely that impotence in diabetes results from four broad causes:
1 Atheroma of the pelvic vessels.
2 Neuropathy affecting smooth-muscle contraction in the walls of arterioles and venules in the corpora cavernosa.
3 Changes in distribution of ions (sodium, potassium, calcium) across the walls of smooth-muscle cells.
4 Psychosocial factors.
Impotence is more common in the elderly, but can occur in young people within a very few years of the onset of the disease — even before there is evidence of more obvious vasculopathy or neuropathy. It has been shown that young men with diabetes who drink alcohol to excess are more likely to develop impotence than those who do not.

Treatment

Treatments are discussed in Chapter 11. Intracavernosal injections of the vaso-dilator papaverine do not work as well in diabetics, possibly because of the greater prevalence of vascular disease.

Liver

Many people with Type II diabetes have fatty infiltration of the liver and mildly abnormal liver function tests.

Skin

Infection

Infection of the skin and mucous membranes is more common in diabetes. This may be tinea or dermatophyte infestation of the skin, nails or toe clefts, or genital candidiasis.

Necrobiosis lipoidica diabeticorum

Necrobiosis is a granulomatous disease which nearly always affects the front of the shins. The skin is red and atrophic (unlike erythema nodosum and pretibial myxoedema, which are raised patches). It is usually non-tender (unlike erythema nodosum). It may appear before the diabetes is diagnosed. Once established it persists, and can be very disfiguring.

Granuloma annulare

Granuloma annulare occurs as small lumpy swellings, often of the forearms and hands. It is histologically very similar to necrobiosis. It is of no clinical significance and is untreatable.

Joints

Cheiroarthropathy

The glycosylation of protein results in the collagen of connective tissue being less distensible than normal. People who have had diabetes from childhood are often unable to stretch their fingers straight.

Frozen shoulder

Frozen shoulder is more common in diabetes. Contraction of the fibrous tissue of the shoulder capsule reduces the joint space, allowing the head of the humerus to rub painfully on the glenoid. It responds well to intra-articular injections of hydrocortisone.

Osteoarthritis

Exuberant osteophytosis of the spine, with occasional anterior fusion, is called Forrestier's disease or diffuse idiopathic skeletal hyperostosis (DISH), and is more common in diabetes.

Diabetic eye disease

After 30 years of diabetes, 12% of Type I diabetics and 5% of Type II diabetics will have lost their sight. However, these data were derived from people diagnosed, and treated, 40 years ago. The number of Type I diabetics who go blind is falling progressively: it used to be 30% at 30 years. However, diabetes is still the commonest cause of blindness under age 60. Cataract is the other main threat to vision.

Cataract

Cataract means opacity of the lens. Cataracts may be central (nuclear) or cortical. Cortical lens opacities may be diffuse or concentrated as spots, lines or spokes. Some lens opacity can be found in 30% of diabetics, especially those who are older. It is of no clinical significance in the majority.

Retinopathy

The main cause of retinopathy is diabetic damage to the capillaries of the retina, leading to ischaemia. Affected retinal capillaries have the following abnormalities:
1 Basement membrane thickening, with defective transfer of nutrients.
2 Saccular aneurysms of their walls (visible on ophthalmoscopy as 'dots').
3 Bleeding from saccular aneurysms ('blots').
4 Exudation ('hard exudates').
5 Thrombosis and obliteration.
The response of the ischaemic retina is to release an unidentified polypeptide angiogenesis factor in an attempt to form new vessels to overcome the ischaemia. When new vessels occur, the person is said to have proliferative retinopathy. The new vessels grow in an uncoordinated way: they are friable and may bleed. Massive haemorrhage causes sudden loss of sight, but it can clear again. Recurrent massive haemorrhage causes blindness. Sometimes the haemorrhage results in fibrous scarring, and this can cause retinal detachment. This sequence of events is the explanation for the different types of retinopathy seen in diabetes:

1   *Background retinopathy:* dots and blots, with hard exudates (accumulation of lipid-rich debris within macrophages).

2   *Maculopathy:* this means background retinopathy affecting the macula. If the macula is affected, vision may be impaired. Maculopathy may also refer to macular oedema — a rare problem resulting from increased transudation.

3   *Preproliferative retinopathy:* a number of changes in the retina suggest that new vessels are about to develop. Oedema of the nerve sheaths appears as ill-defined white patches like summer clouds (cottonwool spots, previously called 'soft exudates'). The veins become distended and irregular in diameter.

4   *Proliferative retinopathy:* new vessels grow from veins, not arterioles. They are visible as leashes of new capillaries, with or without associated haemorrhage.

Treatment of retinopathy

Photocoagulation (laser treatment)

Laser photocoagulation is designed to cause localized destruction of the retina. Multiple burns are made with highly focused laser beams. The objective is the destruction of leaky vessels — those causing hard exudates — and of those likely to bleed, as in proliferative retinopathy. In preproliferative disease the destruction of multiple areas of peripheral retina can cause regression of the changes, presumably by destroying the ischaemic retina which is secreting the angiogenesis factor.

It should be remembered that photocoagulation is a destructive process. It does not restore vision, but hopefully prevents future serious deterioration.

Vitrectomy

Following a single or repeated major haemorrhages the vitreous may be opaque. It is now possible to extract the opaque vitreous and laser the retina under direct vision, and also to reattach any retina which is detached. It can cause miraculous restoration of vision in people who have otherwise been rendered blind. It also sometimes fails.

Neuropathies

Causes

Occlusion of the vasa nervorum results in ischaemic damage to the nerves. The accumulation of toxic metabolites such as sorbitol contributes to this deterioration. A nerve which is affected by these processes is more liable to injury by compression. Hence foot drop (from pressure on the lateral popliteal nerve as it winds around the neck of the fibula) and the carpal tunnel syndrome are more common in diabetes. A classification based on clinical criteria is shown in Table 8.11.

Somatic sensory neuropathy

This is the commonest form of diabetic neuropathy, affecting approximately 30%, especially the elderly. Both large myelinated (soft touch, vibration sense) and

Table 8.11. Neuropathies and neuromyopathies in diabetes

Somatic
Sensory
Motor
Mononeuropathies:
   Amyotrophy
   Truncal radiculopathies
   Cranial nerve palsies

Autonomic
Classical
Heart
Eye
Foot
Penis

Compression neuropathies
Carpal tunnel syndrome
Ulnar compression
Lateral popliteal compression

Spinal cord
Pseudotabes

---

small fibres (myelinated and unmyelinated: pain and temperature) may be affected. The longest fibres are most affected: those to the feet (stocking anaesthesia). Damage is symmetrical.

Although vibration sense is the first detectable abnormality, it is loss of pinprick and pain sensation that are of clinical importance. Someone who cannot feel pain is at greater risk of traumatic injury to the foot. Spontaneous burning sensations (like nettle-sting) — so-called 'painful' neuropathy — are also common, and can cause great distress. Other people complain of cold feet. Sometimes their feet are cold to the touch, and sometimes not. The sensation of coldness results from a combination of neuropathy and vasculopathy.

Somatic motor neuropathy

Like somatic sensory neuropathy this is diffuse and symmetrical, affecting the longer nerves first. In the foot it causes loss of ankle jerk, but this is so common in the general population that it is of little clinical value. Loss of innervation of the muscles which maintain the plantar arch results in one of two deformities: either a flat foot, or one with an exaggerated plantar arch. Both put the foot at risk by causing abnormal pressure distribution.

Severe motor neuropathy will also affect the hands with wasting of the interossei leading to weakness and clumsiness. Motor neuropathy also presents with 'restless legs' — the person's legs jerk for no reason, often when in bed.

Mononeuropathies

Amyotrophy

This is painful, tender wasting and weakness of the muscles of one or both thighs. It affects the quadriceps, hamstrings and gluteals. It may be a presenting symptom of diabetes. It is usually self-limiting, but it may take a year or so before it improves. It improves with better control of blood sugar.

Truncal radiculopathy

This usually presents with pain in the distribution of a dermatome.

Cranial nerve palsy

Isolated dysfunction of one of the cranial nerves (usually the 6th or 3rd) causing ophthalmoplegia (with/without ptosis) is quite common. The reason is unknown. It nearly always settles completely in a few weeks. Involvement of the 3rd nerve (oculomotor) is often painful.

Autonomic neuropathies

Classical autonomic neuropathy

This is the term given to the syndrome which is caused by combined loss of parasympathetic and sympathetic function, with associated loss of innervation of the gastrointestinal and genitourinary tracts. It is uncommon, and people with it usually have multiple complications of diabetes: renal failure, proliferative retinopathy, peripheral somatic neuropathy, cardiac and peripheral vascular disease. Affected people suffer from:

1 Dizziness — due to loss of sympathetic innervation of peripheral vessels.
2 Gustatory sweating — profuse sweating of the head and neck at the taste, smell or even the thought of food.
3 Nocturnal diarrhoea.
4 Gastroparesis — loss of contraction of the stomach, resulting in persistent nausea.
5 Impotence — people with classic autonomic neuropathy are invariably impotent, but many more people have impotence than have classic autonomic neuropathy (see pp. 195–8).
6 Sudden death — presumably from respiratory arrest, or cardiac arrhythmia.

Vagal denervation of the heart

This happens as part of normal ageing, but is more common in diabetes. There is loss of vagally mediated sinus arrhythmia (slowing of the pulse when breathing out).

Autonomic neuropathy and the eye

The pupil normally gets smaller as people get older: the result of reduced sympathetic innervation. There is associated loss of parasympathetic innervation of the eye in old age, and both of these are more common in diabetes.

Autonomic neuropathy and the foot

The foot may be dry from reduced sweating, and the skin is likely to become fissured and infected.

Loss of innervation of the arterioles and venules results in the abnormal shunting of blood in the foot. In extreme cases blood pulses from small arteries to veins but shortcircuits the capillaries. The dorsalis pedis and posterior tibial pulses are easily felt (pounding) and the veins are distended. The foot feels warm, but the superficial tissues are ischaemic. The 'warm ischaemic' foot of autonomic neuropathy is very much at risk.

Autonomic neuropathy and the penis

The physiology of normal erection is not understood, and nor is the pathophysiology of impotence.

Spinal cord

Pseudotabes

Signs of dorsal column loss can complicate diabetes, but the syndrome is very rare. The signs are the same as those of tabes dorsalis complicating tertiary syphilis: loss of vibration sense and deep pain, stamping gait and loss of unconscious proprioception (positive Romberg's sign).

Abnormal function of leucocytes

Abnormal phagocytosis and killing of ingested organisms has been demonstrated in neutrophils and monocytes from people with diabetes. This leads to increased susceptibility to infection by bacteria, yeasts and fungi. The defect is dependent of blood glucose control: there is no increased risk of infection in well-controlled diabetes.

Foot problems in diabetes

Most people find the word 'gangrene', the condition it describes and its treatment by amputation, horrifying. However, amputation is only rarely necessary. The people most at risk are the elderly (often Type II), and younger diabetics who smoke cigarettes.

Causes of foot problems

Foot problems occur only in those whose feet are 'at risk'. The reasons why the feet of any one diabetic may be at risk are listed in Table 8.12.

The single factor which precipitates ulceration or gangrene in an 'at risk' foot is a break in the skin. Once the skin becomes broken, bacteria can enter the tissues.

The neuropathic foot

Motor neuropathy alters the shape of the plantar arch, causing increased pressure — usually over the metatarsal heads, the knuckles and the tips of the toes. The person feels no pain because he or she has sensory neuropathy. The increased pressure causes a build-up of hard skin (callus), and this increases the

Table 8.12. Factors which render a foot 'at risk' in diabetes

---

Ischaemia
Large-vessel disease — atherosclerosis
Abnormal small-vessel circulation from autonomic denervation
Capillary abnormalities

Sensory neuropathy
Anaesthesia

Motor neuropathy
Increased pressure

Autonomic neuropathy
Abnormal microcirculation
Charcot foot
Reduced sweating; altered skin integrity and resistance to infection

Abnormal leucocyte function
Hyperglycaemia increases risk of infection

Poor eyesight and ageing
Neglect of feet; inability to cut nails

---

pressure further. The pressure causes necrosis under the callus and the skin breaks down, leaving a clean, punched-out 'neuropathic' ulcer. These lesions are treated by keeping them clean with daily dressings, and taking the pressure off the affected area. Fitted footwear prevents recurrence.

The ischaemic foot

Whereas the skin of the neuropathic foot looks rather puffy, pale and thick, the skin of an ischaemic foot is thin, red and glassy. The skin might be broken as a result of any injury, and the likelihood of injury is increased if there is associated neuropathy.

When the skin is broken bacteria enter the tissues, causing cellulitis. The associated inflammation causes thrombosis of the already narrowed arterioles, and gangrene (black, necrotic tissue) results. There may be gangrene of a toe (which is usually dry and circumscribed) or gangrene of the forefoot (which is usually wet and obviously infected). Some form of amputation is usually inevitable when gangrene occurs. Gangrene is a sign of severe underlying ischaemia.

Angiography should be performed at an early stage to determine whether the blood supply can be improved by angioplasty or bypass surgery.

The neuroischaemic foot

The neuroischaemic foot has thin, red, anaesthetic skin. There may be a clean ulcer over a pressure point, such as a malleolus or the medial aspect of the first metatarsophalangeal joint.

Osteomyelitis

Infection of bone is a relatively uncommon complication of penetrating infection. *Staphylococcus aureus* and anaerobic bacteria are usually responsible.

The infection nearly always affects the metatarsals and phalanges. It usually heals with effective antibiotic therapy after 2–3 months, but many surgeons advocate early drainage, with amputation of the toe.

The Charcot foot

The Charcot foot of diabetes is very different from the Charcot joint (spine, hip or knee) of tertiary syphilis. In syphilis the lesion occurs because there is complete loss of deep pain sensation, and the joint is disorganized by repeated and unheeded trauma. In the Charcot foot of diabetes, deep pain sensation is intact — and the basic problem is dissolution of the bones of the tarsus — probably by increased arteriovenous shunting from autonomic neuropathy. In response to minor trauma, the bones collapse (often painfully) and the foot changes shape. If the person does not obtain surgical shoes, the skin will ulcerate over pressure points.

Heel ulcers

Big ulcers on the heel occur in ischaemic feet when the person is confined to bed for some reason (pressure sores). Once established they can be impossible to treat. Heel ulcers hardly ever heal.

Small spontaneous ulcers occur on the heels, presumably from end-artery occlusion and ischaemia. Unlike most diabetic foot ulcers, they can be very painful. They are difficult to treat and may persist for months or years.

Critical ischaemia

Diabetics may present with occlusion of a major artery due to thrombosis complicating atherosclerosis, or from arterial embolus. The foot is red (subcritical ischaemia) or white (acute critical ischaemia) and is very painful. If early embolectomy is not possible, amputation is inevitable.

SCREENING FOR COMPLICATIONS OF DIABETES

All people with diabetes should expect to be screened for complications at least annually. Complications should be detected before they become symptomatic. When symptoms occur, it is often too late.

There are four complications which should be specifically sought at routine screening:

1 *Proteinuria:* once proteinuria occurs, the person is at much increased risk of hypertension, vascular disease, retinopathy and renal failure. The diabetic with proteinuria is watched more closely than one without. Plasma urea and creatinine should be checked regularly.

Measurement of microalbuminuria may become established as a routine process in the future.

2 *Blood pressure:* hypertension is treated more aggressively in diabetics than in non-diabetics, especially if they have proteinuria.

3 *Eyes:* screening for change in visual acuity and for retinopathy should be routine in the surgery. Measurement of intraocular pressure by optometrists should be routine in those aged over 55 years.

4 *Feet:* it is usual to recommend annual screening of the feet of all diabetics, but it is doubtful if this is a productive exercise in anyone under the age of 50 unless:

(a) They are known to have vascular disease.

(b) They have symptoms suggesting neuropathy.

(c) They have hypertension, proteinuria, significant retinopathy.

(d) They smoke.

DEFINITION OF MANAGEMENT OBJECTIVES IN DIABETES

The definition of appropriate objectives is the key to the successful management of this complex and potentially awful disease. There is no point in spending hours talking about foot care to a 14-year-old, and there is no point in striving to achieve close blood glucose control in a 78-year-old who is blind and who has had a disabling stroke.

Objectives in the newly diagnosed diabetic have been detailed above. Objectives in the established diabetic fall into five broad groups. Those appropriate to each person should be agreed with them.

1 Relief of symptoms.

2 Prevention of complications — achieving normoglycaemia (education, diet, treatments, monitoring), health-care advice.

3 Screening for complications.

4 Treatment of complications.

5 Treatment of associated problems: obesity, hyperlipidaemia, pregnancy.

Management objectives should be agreed with the patient, and each interview and check should be geared to determining whether or not they have been met. If they have not, and prove unattainable, then different objectives need to be established and agreed.

Thus weight loss might be an obvious initial objective in an obese Type II diabetic, but once he or she demonstrates their inability to lose weight, then secondary objectives should be established. The main priority might then become screening for complications, or simply the management of symptoms.

There is nothing to be gained from repeatedly urging the patient to strive for targets which are patently unattainable — it only leads to frustration and anger on both sides, with alienation and despair. It is more rewarding for everyone to concentrate on objectives which can be achieved.

Chapter 9
Fat and Fat Metabolism

Lipids are not soluble in water: they are carried in blood bound to transport proteins called apoproteins. The complex is known as a lipoprotein. Lipids and lipoproteins are mostly thought of as risk factors for cardiovascular disease, and their physiological function is often overlooked.

LIPIDS

Lipids occur as free (non-esterified) fatty acids, triglycerides, phosholipids and cholesterol.

Free fatty acids

Short-chain fatty acids may circulate free (free, or non-esterified, fatty acids, FFAs or NEFAs) or esterified — either to cholesterol or to glycerol. Whether esterified or not, fatty acids are bound to albumin for transport in the blood. Fatty acids are an essential source of energy in times of starvation, as the body's carbohydrate reserves are small (< 300 kcal) and last for only a few hours. Fat is ideal as an energy store because of

1   its high calorie yield per gram;
2   its reduced requirement for water; and
3   its insulating properties.

FFAs are metabolized by liver and muscle. They may be oxidized, re-esterified or converted to other fatty acids.

Triglycerides

Triglycerides are the main storage form of fatty acids: three acids are esterified into each glycerol molecule. Triglycerides in blood are derived from two main sources: the gut and the liver.

Gut

Absorbed fatty acids and monoglycerides are converted to triglycerides within the small intestine. They are then compounded with lesser amounts of glycerol, phospholipid and apoprotein to form large globular chylomicrons. These pass from the intestinal lymphatics into the blood stream via the thoracic duct.

Liver

Triglycerides synthesized within the liver are released into the blood stream as rather smaller lipoprotein complexes — very low-density lipoproteins (VLDLs). Over 90% of circulating triglycerides are absorbed: 80–170 mmol, 70–150 g day^{-1}. Absorbed triglycerides are cleared from the blood within 12 hours, and hence concentrations in a fasting sample reflect endogenous synthesis.

Phospholipids

Phospholipids are made by all cells, but those in the circulation come mainly from the liver. The principal circulating forms are sphyngomyelin and phosphatidylcholine (lecithin). Phospholipids are an integral part of cell membranes, and serve as precursors for many important substances: arachidonic acid derivatives (thromboxane, prostacyclin) and intracellular second messengers (diacylglycerol and inositol triphosphate) (see Figs 1.12, 1.14 and 1.15). Phospholipids also help render triglycerides and cholesterol soluble by combining with them in lipoproteins.

Cholesterol

Cholesterol may be free or esterified (principally to the fatty acids oleate and linoleate). It is an integral part of cell membranes and contributes to their plasticity. It is also the precursor for the bile acid synthesis which is essential for the absorption of fat and fat-soluble substances from the gut. Cholesterol is the precursor for the synthesis of steroid hormones — glucocorticoids, mineralocorticoids and sex steroids.

Although most cells have the capacity to synthesize cholesterol, they tend to utilize that which is in the circulation. Circulating cholesterol is either absorbed or synthesized by the liver. The rate-limiting step in cholesterol synthesis is the conversion of acetate to mevalonic acid by the enzyme 3-hydroxy-3-methylglutaryl coenzyme A reductase.

Principles of lipid metabolism

Fatty acids and triglycerides are concerned with the storage and provision of energy. FFAs are derived from the diet (exogenous lipid pathway, Fig. 9.1) or from VLDL secreted by the liver (endogenous pathway, Fig. 9.2). Excess FFAs are stored as triglycerides in fat cells.

Phospholipids and cholesterol are the principal components of cell membranes and act as precursors for important biologically active substances. Choles-

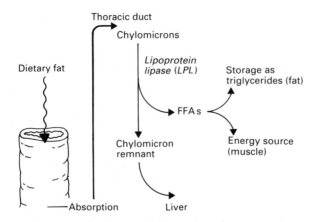

Fig. 9.1. Exogenous lipid pathway (metabolism of dietary fat). FFA, free fatty acids.

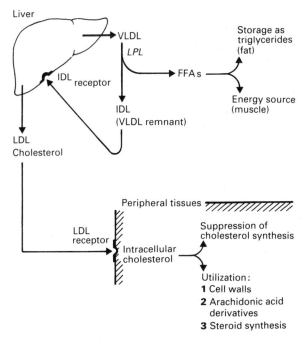

Fig. 9.2. Endogenous lipid pathway. IDL, LDL and VLDL, intermediate, low and very low density lipoproteins.

terol is synthesized by most cells, but circulating cholesterol is mainly derived from the liver (endogenous lipid pathway).

There is a finite amount of cholesterol with which cells can deal. There are no intracellular stores of cholesterol. When cells are saturated, the cell-surface

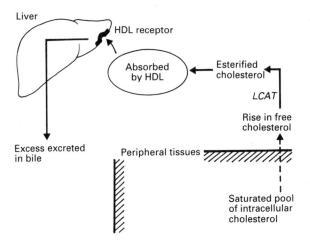

Fig. 9.3. Reverse cholesterol pathway — the protective action of HDL (high density lipoprotein). LCAT, lecithin-cholesterol acyltransferase.

receptors for cholesterol are down-regulated and intracellular synthesis is halted. When cholesterol is not taken up by the tissues, the concentration of cholesterol in blood rises. It is esterified and absorbed by high-density lipoprotein (HDL). HDL is thus a cholesterol scavenger (reverse cholesterol pathway, Fig. 9.3). HDL cholesterol is returned to the liver and excess is excreted in the bile.

APOPROTEINS

Apoproteins render cholesterol and triglycerides transportable in blood by incorporating them into lipoproteins. Apoproteins are helical structures with lipophilic inner, and hydrophilic outer, surfaces — they wrap around the lipids they transport. Apoproteins also interact with target organ binding sites and facilitate the entry of lipids into cells. They may also act as cofactors (e.g. apo CII is a cofactor for lipoprotein lipase). There are a large number of them but the principal ones are listed in Table 9.1.

Table 9.1. Apoproteins

Apoprotein	Size	Comment
Apo AI	17 kDa	Cofactor for LCAT
Apo AII	28 kDa	With apo AI is main binding protein of HDL
Apo B100	512 kDa	Major apoprotein of LDL
Apo B48	240 kDa	Structurally identical to N-terminal 48 amino acids of B100. Only found in chylomicrons
Apo CI, CII, CIII	6–9 kDa	CII is a cofactor for LPL
Apo E	34 kDa	In VLDL, IDL and HDL Facilitates cholesterol transfer between blood and tissues

LCAT, lecithin cholesterol acyl transferase; VLDL, LDL, IDL, HDL, very low, low, intermediate and high density lipoproteins.

LIPOPROTEINS

The basic structure of lipoproteins is shown in Fig. 9.4. Compounds with ionic groups (and hence relatively hydrophilic) are ranged around the shell — phospholipids, unesterified cholesterol and proteins. In the centre droplets of non-polar lipids, triglycerides and esterified cholesterol are wrapped in apoproteins. Lipoproteins are classified according to their sizes, as determined by ultracentrifugation, into chylomicrons (the least dense), VLDL, IDL, LDL and HDL (the most dense).

Chylomicrons

Chylomicrons are formed in the cells of the small intestine and are used for transporting absorbed fats into the circulation. Ninety per cent of the fat is triglyceride. They are 10–20 times bigger than any other lipoprotein. Chylomicrons are normally cleared from the blood within 12 hours of a meal.

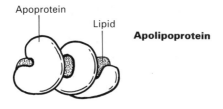

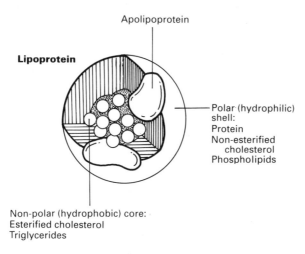

Fig. 9.4. The structure of lipoproteins.

VLDL

Very low-density lipoproteins are synthesized in the liver and are the medium for transporting triglycerides to the periphery for storage. They also act as precursors for the formation of LDL, which is the main cholesterol transport. VLDL synthesis increases in response to an increase in circulating FFAs and carbohydrate.

IDL

Intermediate-density lipoproteins are also called VLDL remnants. They are converted to LDL in the liver.

LDL

Low-density lipoproteins are formed from VLDL by the action of the enzyme lipoprotein lipase (LPL) which is sited on endothelial cells. Lipoprotein lipase cleaves the bulk of the triglyceride from the VLDL, leaving IDL (VLDL remnant; see Fig. 9.2). IDL is converted to LDL in the liver. LDL interacts with LDL receptors on target tissues, and the receptor–LDL complex is taken into the cell. The receptor is recycled, the apoprotein is degraded and the cholesterol is available for utilization. When the cell is saturated with cholesterol, its own endogenous synthesis is inhibited and the cell-surface receptors for LDL are down-regulated.

HDL

High-density lipoproteins are more dense because they contain a much greater percentage of apoprotein compared with lipid (Table 9.2). There are two main forms, HDL2 and HDL3, and they are derived from both gut and liver. HDL3 is converted to HDL2 by the action of the enzyme lecithin–cholesterol acyltransferase (LCAT) which transfers esterified cholesterol to the lipoprotein (see below). HDLs function as cholesterol scavengers, transporting excess cholesterol from peripheral tissues to the liver. For this reason HDL is cardioprotective: people with higher levels are at less risk of cardiovascular disease.

Factors affecting lipoprotein metabolism

Enzymes involved in lipoprotein metabolism

LPL

Lipoprotein lipases are bound to the endothelial cells. They act on triglyceride-rich chylomicrons and VLDL. Women have more LPL activity than men. Exercise increases LPL activity in muscle endothelium; ethanol increases LPL activity in fat. LPL is stimulated by insulin, and activity is therefore reduced in diabetes mellitus. LPL bound to hepatic endothelium is called hepatic lipase: it converts IDL to LDL.

LCAT

Lecithin–cholesterol acyltransferase is responsible for transferring esterified cholesterol to and from lipoproteins.

HMG CoA reductase

This is the rate-limiting enzyme in cholesterol synthesis.

Congenital abnormalities

Inherited LDL receptor deficiency occurs in familial hypercholesterolaemia (FH). The prevalence of homozygotes is 1 in 1 000 000, but heterozygotes (1 in 500) are also affected.

Constitutional and social factors

Age and sex

The concentration of cholesterol and triglycerides in childhood is about 4.0 and

Table 9.2. Relative constitution of lipoproteins

Lipoprotein	Diameter (nm)	Protein (%)	Triglyceride (%)	Cholesterol (%)
Chylomicron	500–1000	2	90	2
VLDL	80	10	60	20
IDL	40	20	30	40
LDL	20	25	5	50
HDL	5	50	2	15

0.65 mmol litre^{-1}, respectively. Both rise at the time of puberty, and the concentration of HDL in boys falls. There is a slow rise in both cholesterol and triglycerides throughout adult life, unrelated to obesity. After the menopause the concentration of HDL is equal in the two sexes.

Pregnancy

Hypercholesterolaemia and hypertriglyceridaemia may be caused by increased apoprotein synthesis induced by oestrogens.

Race

There may be some racial differences, but much of the observed difference in the incidence of heart disease in different countries is related to diet.

Exercise

Moderate exercise induces increases in muscle LPL, with a progressive reduction in triglycerides and LDL cholesterol, with a rise in HDL3.

Smoking

Serum triglyceride concentration is proportional to nicotine intake.

Dietary factors

Obesity

Excessive caloric intake causes obesity. This causes a rise in VLDL (mainly triglycerides) and a fall in cardioprotective HDL. These may be caused by insulin resistance secondary to the obesity.

Carbohydrate

Increased intake of refined carbohydrate (e.g. glucose, sucrose) causes increased hepatic synthesis of triglycerides.

Fat

Intake of saturated fatty acids (meat and dairy products) has a greater adverse effect on lipoprotein metabolism than intake of cholesterol, with reduced HDL levels and increased LDL. Preferential intake of polyunsaturated fats (vegetable oils) reduces LDL, but also reduces HDL.

Monounsaturated fats (oleate in olive oil) reduce LDL but leave HDL unchanged. Cardiac disease is low in Mediterranean countries, where the intake of olive oil is high.

Fat people need to reduce total fat intake because of its calorific value. A low-fat diet is not particularly good for lean people, however, because they will tend to make up their calorie intake with carbohydrate, which may increase hepatic triglyceride synthesis.

Protein

There is some evidence that non-animal protein, such as soya bean protein, is also beneficial.

Fibre
>   Increased intake of dietary fibre displaces other nutrients from the meal, and thus tends to lower serum LDL and triglycerides.

Ethanol
>   Alcohol has a protective effect, unless it is taken to excess. It increases HDL2 and HDL3 — possibly by stimulating LPL. Excessive intake causes hypertriglyceridaemia.

Coffee
>   Excessive coffee drinking increases serum cholesterol. This is unrelated to caffeine, because it does not happen with instant coffee.

Drugs

Oral contraceptives
>   Women taking the combined (oestrogen plus progestogen) preparations have higher serum cholesterol and triglycerides than normal. In addition, most progestogens (desogestrel is an exception) are effectively androgenic and may suppress HDL. Women who are at risk of cardiac disease should probably not take oral contraceptives, unless — possibly — they contain non-androgenic progestogens.

Hormone replacement therapy
>   Oestrogen therapy after the menopause seems to be largely beneficial — by increasing serum HDL. There is no logical reason why women at risk of cardiac disease should be denied hormone replacement therapy, unless there is some other specific contraindication.

Thiazides
>   Thiazide diuretics increase triglycerides and cholesterol (VLDL and LDL), but have no effect on HDL.

β-Blockers
>   β-Blockers may increase serum triglycerides by up to 30%, and may also suppress HDL. These effects of thiazides and β-blockers may be one reason why the treatment of mild to moderate hypertension has never been shown to reduce the risk of myocardial infarction.

Glucocorticoids
>   Glucocorticoids induce insulin resistance, with hypertriglyceridaemia and reduced HDL.

Cyclosporin
>   Cyclosporin raises LDL cholesterol.

Hyperlipoproteinaemia secondary to other conditions
>   Hyperlipoproteinaemia can occur in a number of other diseases, often as a result of malnutrition or defective insulin action (Table 9.3).

Table 9.3. Secondary hyperlipidaemias. N, normal

Condition	Triglyceride	Cholesterol	Lipoprotein
Anorexia nervosa	N	+	LDL
Hypothyroidism	N	+	LDL
Type I diabetes	+	N	Chylomicron, VLDL
Type II diabetes	+	N	VLDL
Renal diseases	+	+	VLDL, LDL
Liver diseases	+	+	VLDL, LDL
Gout	+	N	VLDL
Ethanol	+	N	Chylomicron, VLDL

Anorexia nervosa

There is gross elevation of LDL. This may be partly a starvation effect and partly the effect of abnormal diet.

Hypothyroidism

Hypercholesterolaemia (LDL) is the commonest consequence. It has been suggested that 20% of women over age 40 with hypercholesterolaemia will be hypothyroid.

Insulin-dependent (Type I) diabetes

In untreated insulin-dependent diabetes, LPL deficiency causes FFA release, and this stimulates hepatic triglyceride synthesis. Gross hypertriglyceridaemia is one reason why diabetic ketoacidosis may present with acute pancreatitis.

Non-insulin-dependent (Type II) diabetes

Hyperglycaemia causes increased hepatic triglyceride synthesis. There may be some LPL deficiency with increased FFA release as well. HDL is reduced.

Renal disease

In the nephrotic syndrome, serum albumin concentrations are reduced as a result of renal loss. Hypoalbuminaemia results in increased availability of FFAs, and these stimulate VLDL (and hence LDL) synthesis. Hypertriglyceridaemia is common also in those on dialysis.

Liver disease

Hypoalbuminaemia may cause hyperlipoproteinaemia, as in the nephrotic syndrome. In addition, hyperlipidaemia occurs in obstructive jaundice, stimulated by the reabsorption of biliary lecithin.

Gout

Hypertriglyceridaemia occurs in 30% — possibly related to ethanol, obesity or thiazides.

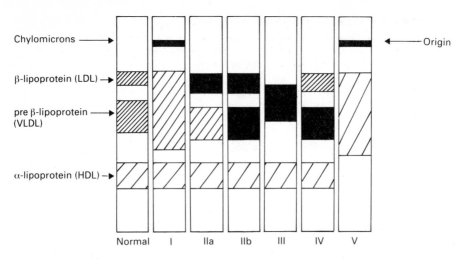

Fig. 9.5. Agarose gel electrophoresis of lipoproteins. Diagrammatic representation of the electrophoretic pattern seen in different hyperlipidaemias (Frederickson classification).

Abnormalities of lipoprotein metabolism

Six broad categories of hyperlipoproteinaemia are recognized. They are defined on the basis of electrophoretic mobility of the serum lipids (Fig. 9.5). This is the Frederickson classification.

Type I

Deficiency of LPL (or of its cofactor, apo CII) results in inability to clear chylomicrons. The serum is white and fatty to the naked eye. Total cholesterol is elevated, and triglycerides markedly so.

Type IIa

Inherited deficiency of the LDL receptor results in high LDL cholesterol — FH. Homozygotes die of myocardial infarction at an early age. Heterozygotes are also at risk of early cardiovascular disease, but are treatable. Type IIa can complicate untreated hypothyroidism.

Type IIb

There is increased LDL and VLDL (mixed triglycerides and cholesterol). The inherited form is called familial combined hyperlipoproteinaemia. Type IIb can also complicate diabetes, renal failure and anorexia nervosa.

Type III

Failure to clear chylomicron remnants and IDL may result from a deficiency of hepatic lipase. It may be familial, or it may be secondary to obesity or diabetes.

Table 9.4. Clinical classification of hyperlipidaemias

Common (polygenic) hypercholesterolaemia (Frederickson Type IIa)
Slight increase in total cholesterol and slight increase in CHD risk

Familial combined hyperlipoproteinaemia (Frederickson IIb, or IV)
Slight increase in cholesterol and in triglyceride. Moderate CHD risk

FH (Frederickson IIa)
Gross hypercholesterolaemia, with greatly increased risk of CHD

Remnant hyperlipoproteinaemia (Frederickson III)
Gross hypercholesterolaemia and triglyceridaemia. Greatly increased risk of CHD

Hyperchylomicronaemia (Frederickson I or V)
Gross hypertriglyceridaemia, with great risk of pancreatitis

Familial hypertriglyceridaemia (Frederickson Type IV or V)
Hypertriglyceridaemia with increased risk of pancreatitis, and probably of CHD

CHD, coronary heart disease.

Type IV

The main abnormality is high serum VLDL levels, affecting especially triglycerides. Familial forms occurs, but Type IV can be caused by diabetes or renal failure.

Type V

Type V is a mixture of Types I and IV. It can be the result of inherited apo CII deficiency, but is usually caused by alcohol, β-blockers, thiazides or oral contraceptives. An alternative classification is shown in Table 9.4.

Clinical manifestations of hyperlipidaemia

Corneal arcus

A normal feature of ageing, but may be associated with hyperlipoproteinaemia in young people.

Xanthelasmata

Associated with hyperlipoproteinaemia in approximately 50% of cases.

Tendon xanthomata

These are fatty lumps adjacent to tendon sheaths (particularly hands and Achilles tendon), and occur most commonly in FH.

Eruptive xanthomata

Widespread, irritating eruptions which are associated with gross hypertriglyceridaemia, especially in familial forms.

THE PATHOGENESIS OF ATHEROSCLEROSIS

Atherosclerosis involves changes in both the intima and the media of arterial walls. The changes are partly caused by metabolic defects, and partly by physical ones.

The accumulation of lipids within the walls is probably caused by hyperlipidaemia, with fat-filled monocytes passing from the circulation through the endothelium. Atherosclerosis is extremely uncommon if total serum cholesterol is less than 4.0 mmol litre^{-1}. However, other processes are involved: smooth-muscle cell proliferation occurs, probably stimulated by platelet-derived growth factor (PDGF). Other growth factors, e.g. falling insulin-like growth factor (IGF_1), may contribute to the loss of elastin which occurs, and the increasing fibrosis. Hyperinsulinaemia from insulin resistance — both in obesity and in Type II diabetes — has been implicated, as has free radical generation within the endothelium.

Hypertension accelerates atherogenesis, due to a presumed physical effect on the intima: atheroma is more common at sites in the aorta subjected to maximal pressure.

The next phase of the disease is characterized by interruption of the intima over the atheromatous patch. This may be precipitated by the growth of smooth-muscle cells, or by blood-borne irritants: carbon monoxide (smoking), viruses, or LDL itself. Once the intima is breached, thrombus forms on the bared tissue and causes vascular occlusion.

Cardiovascular risk factors

Serum cholesterol

There is no upper limit of normal in serum cholesterol: the increased risk of coronary heart disease is continuous. Nevertheless, the risk rises exponentially (Fig. 9.6). Half of all cardiovascular deaths occur in those with serum cholesterol concentrations above the 85th centile (6.5 mmol litre^{-1}).

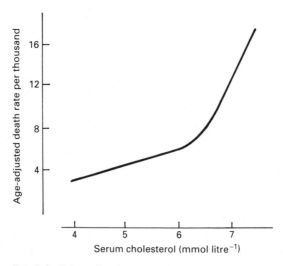

Fig. 9.6. Relationship between serum cholesterol and heart disease in men.

Triglycerides

Hypertriglyceridaemia is associated with increased risk, independent of other factors. The mechanism is not clear.

Reduced HDL

High-density lipoprotein is protective: lower levels are associated with increased risk. As in the case of cholesterol the relationship is continuous, with no clear cut-off between normal and abnormal. However, those with concentrations of HDL < 0.9 mmol litre^{-1} are especially at risk. The increased risk of heart disease in men may be attributed to the suppressive effect of androgens on HDL synthesis.

Age

The risks of heart disease and stroke increase markedly with age.

Sex

Younger men are three times more likely to have a heart attack than premenopausal women of the same age and the same serum cholesterol.

Blood pressure

Hypertension doubles the risk (even though lowering high blood pressure has never been proved to reduce it).

Smoking

Smoking almost doubles the risk. Hypertensive people who smoke are especially liable. A normotensive, non-smoking 45-year-old man with a cholesterol of 5 mmol litre^{-1} has a 2% risk of developing coronary heart disease in the next 8 years, compared with a 20% risk in a 45-year-old cigarette-smoker with hypertension and a cholesterol of 8 mmol litre^{-1}.

MANAGEMENT OF HYPERLIPOPROTEINAEMIA

Management is geared towards reducing the serum lipoprotein concentration, and hence (hopefully) to reducing the risk of vascular disease. The choice of treatment must be determined by the chances of achieving success. Priorities need to be established: stopping smoking and weight reduction are far more likely to improve the prognosis than drugs (either for hyperlipoproteinaemia or for hypertension). However, recent data from the Framingham Study suggests that obese people who lose weight and then regain it may have a worse cardiovascular mortality than those who never lose weight at all. In this case it is reasonable to assume that it was the regain in weight which was harmful, rather than the initial dieting.

Drugs should be prescribed as an adjunct to diet, not as an alternative. Drugs which are shown to be ineffective (for whatever reason) should not be continued. Drugs which lower serum cholesterol increase the incidence of gallstones, and some may also increase the risk of carcinoma of the gastrointestinal tract. Indeed, all major trials of lipid-lowering therapy have hitherto produced the same general result: reduced deaths from cardiovascular disease, but no change in death rate overall. All have shown the same — totally unexplained — increase in violent death (accidents, suicide etc.). Until this is explained, it is felt that aggressive lipid-lowering therapy should be reserved for high-risk groups.

The main benefit of defining hyperlipoproteinaemia in an older person presenting with, for example, a myocardial infarction, may be that it will lead to the detection of a familial condition affecting his or her children. The earlier treatment is instituted, the more likely it is to work.

Education

The reasons for treatment should be explained, and both doctor and patient should agree desirable end-points. The risks of treatment, especially of drugs, should also be explained. The significance of obesity and of cigarettes needs to be put in perspective. Young women should be advised about the potential risks of combined (oestrogen and progesterone) contraceptives.

Diet

Fat people should reduce their calorie intake and try to lose weight. This usually involves a reduction in total fat intake. Those who lose weight should be encouraged to stay thinner. Thin people should not reduce total fat but should preferentially increase their intake of vegetable fats (NB: coconut oil is an important exception — it contains more saturated fat than most animal sources. Non-specific 'vegetable oils' on supermarket shelves may well contain coconut oil.) Meat from fish or chicken will contain less saturated fat than meat from other animals. Reduced intake of refined carbohydrate will reduce triglycerides, and oils from fatty fish (e.g. mackerel or herring) will increase HDL. Olive oil reduces LDL.

Drugs for hypertriglyceridaemia

These drugs generally lower triglycerides by up to 30%, and there is usually an associated small reduction in cholesterol.

Fibrates

Clofibrate was the first to be introduced, but has been mainly replaced by bezafibrate and gemfibrizol. They are particularly valuable in the hypertriglyceridaemia which complicates diabetes. As they are protein-bound in blood, they displace sulphonylureas and enhance their hypoglycaemic potency. They also enhance the potency of warfarin. The most serious side-effect is (reversible) myositis — which is most likely in people with renal disease.

Nicotinic acid and derivatives

These work by reducing VLDL synthesis and increasing HDL. Flushing is the main side-effect, but it can be reduced by taking the nicotinic acid with meals, or after aspirin.

Fish oils

The long-chain polyunsaturated fatty acids in fish oil can cause a marked reduction in both triglycerides and cholesterol. Preparations of fish oils in capsules are expensive, however, and as much may be achieved by appropriate dietary advice.

Drugs for hypercholesterolaemia

Anion exchange resins

These bind bile acids in the gut and prevent their reabsorption. Examples are cholestyramine (up to 24 g daily) and colestipol (10 g b.d.). When taken long-term they reduce LDL cholesterol by over 10%, and raise HDL by 3%. They are especially suitable for children with heterozygous FH, because of their safety. Unfortunately, many people stop taking them because of gastrointestinal side-effects, especially constipation.

Probucol

This causes a 10–20% reduction in cholesterol by an unknown mechanism.

HMG CoA reductase inhibitors

Three which have been marketed are lovastatin, pravastatin and simvastatin. They inhibit endogenous cholesterol synthesis, and this also has the effect of increasing the expression of the cell-surface LDL receptor, and extracting LDL cholesterol from serum. They work well in heterozygous FH, but not in homozygotes (who are unable to generate LDL receptors at all). They are better at reducing LDL cholesterol than fibrates, but less effective on triglycerides. Like fibrates they also cause myositis, and the two drugs should only be used in combination with great care — especially in renal failure, or in those taking cyclosporin.

OBESITY

People who are overweight have increased amounts of triglyceride stored as fat. People who are 10–20% above the upper limit of the range for ideal body weight are called 'overweight'. Those greater than 20% over are 'obese'. The concept of small-, medium- and large-frame people is now discarded. The Quettelet index or body mass index (BMI; $kg\,m^{-2}$) is used increasingly: normal is 20–25; overweight 25–28; obese > 28.

Effects of obesity

Overweight and obese people have between 1.25 and 2.5 times the risk of developing hypertensive, cardiovascular and biliary tract disease. The risk of stroke is increased only slightly in frank obesity. Other medical complications include an increased predisposition to Type II diabetes, osteoarthritis, varicose veins and anaesthetic hazards. The most common consequences of obesity are psychological and social, at least in western societies: loss of self-esteem, self-consciousness, social isolation, frustration and depression.

Pathogenesis

The causes of obesity are multiple, and vary from person to person. Although many fat people undoubtedly overeat, it is likely that some, at least, are metabolically different from their lean counterparts. However, it should be remembered that a person has to ingest 2000 kcal daily simply to maintain a body mass of 100 kg (16 stones).

Adipocyte metabolism

Fat cells are essential for the continuous supply of energy (FFAs) in an organism such as a human, that feeds only intermittently. This was particularly true when humans were opportunist hunters and gatherers, and the interval between meals must have been greater than it is today. The body stores only about 300 kcal in the form of glycogen, and energy supplies are dependent on lipolysis as soon as carbohydrate reserves are exhausted.

This lipolysis is catalysed by hormone-sensitive lipase (HSL). HSL is activated by some hormones which stimulate cAMP production — ACTH, catecholamines (β-receptors), glucagon — and inhibited by insulin.

Insulin secretion is suppressed when carbohydrate reserves are low, and this allows the lysis of stored triglyceride by HSL. This occurs normally in fasting.

In contrast, feeding results in a rise in blood sugar and in insulin. The insulin inhibits HSL, thereby preventing lipolysis. Insulin also increases triglyceride formation in the adipocyte by

1 stimulating LPL, which releases fatty acids from VLDL, and

2 stimulating glucose uptake, which acts as precursor for the formation of glycerol phosphate, the precursor of triglyceride synthesis.

Regional variation in adipocytes

Different fat cells have quantitatively different functions. The cells on the abdomen are more sensitive to β-adrenergic stimulation than the cells on the thigh. This means that they undergo lipolysis more readily, with increased FFA release. Overweight men tend to develop truncal obesity, while women develop fatter thighs and buttocks, and this may explain why overweight men are more at risk of cardiovascular disease, because the increased abdominal fat is more likely to release FFAs. Thus the obesity of men is more likely to be associated with hyperlipoproteinaemia. For this reason the 'waist–hip ratio' has been described as an added indicator of cardiovascular risk.

These metabolic differences are not invariable. Other changes take place, for example, in pregnancy: the adipocytes of the thigh develop reduced HSL activity and lipolysis is increased, making FFAs available for milk synthesis.

Adipocyte size and adipocyte number

It has been suggested that overfeeding in the neonatal period may stimulate the differentiation of a larger number of adipocytes, and that the individual with more fat cells is more likely to become obese. Fat cell numbers also increase at the time of puberty, and it is possible that a similar process takes place then as well.

There is no doubt that fat people do have larger numbers of fat cells than the non-obese, but it has not been established that this is caused by overfeeding at certain critical periods of development. However, the increased numbers of cells helps explain why fat people have greater difficulty in losing weight by dieting (see below).

Brown adipose tissue

Brown fat is structurally and functionally different from white fat. It is richly innervated by a sympathetic nerve supply which originates in the preoptic and ventromedial areas of the hypothalamus. The cells have many more mitochondria, and the lipid droplets in the cytoplasm are small and multiple rather than single and large. The function of brown adipose tissue (BAT) is heat production, and not FFA storage.

Deposits of brown fat are found between the scapulae of neonates, and around the kidneys, but are otherwise scanty in humans. They may play a part in allowing the newborn baby to cope with the cold stress of being born, but they are probably of greater functional importance in non-primate mammals, particularly ones which hibernate. The thermogenic effect of BAT depends on the intracellular production of thermogenin in response to the action of insulin and carbohydrate. Thermogenin uncouples oxidative phosphorylation, generating heat rather than adenosine triphosphate (ATP).

Triiodothyronine and the adipocyte

Thyroid hormones are probably crucial to the metabolism of both BAT and white fat cells. Thyroid hormones act synergistically with catecholamines and stimulate lipolysis. They antagonize the actions of insulin. It is possible that the effect on fat cells is more dependent on circulating triiodothyronine (T_3) than on thyroxine (T_4), because fat cells do not possess the deiodinase necessary to generate T_3 locally. It is interesting to note that reduced synthesis of hepatic T_3 is one of the endocrine consequences of fasting, and this presumably represents an attempt to conserve fat stores. In thyrotoxicosis BAT cells are depleted.

Response of the adipocyte to obesity and to fasting

The hypertrophic, triglyceride-stretched adipocyte acquires insulin resistance. In an attempt to limit further fat storage it loses the ability to trap FFAs and glucose, and intracellular synthesis of glycerol phosphate from glucose is reduced as well. On the other hand, lipolysis is relatively unopposed. As the intake of calories is reduced, the insulin sensitivity returns and may become exaggerated. The result is that a fat person who is trying to lose weight by dieting will have initial success, but the advantage of insulin insensitivity is lost after a few days. The increased numbers of fat cells in obesity worsens the effect of restored sensitivity.

Metabolic rate in obesity

Basal metabolic rate (BMR) is increased in fat people, and the energy required for simple movements and physical tasks is also increased. The reason for the high BMR is probably the increase in lean body mass which accompanies obesity: 30–50% of BMR is accounted for simply by the activity of Na–K-ATPase. Obese people do, however, have reduced post-prandial thermogenesis. This can be regarded as more 'efficient' use of ingested calories — they are converted to fat rather than squandered as heat.

Furthermore, it was demonstrated in the classic 'Vermont' study (in which volunteers in prison were fed excessive calories and then allowed to regain their former weight) that fat people required only half the energy expenditure to retain their normal fatness, than usually lean people who had acquired fatness by short-term overeating.

Inheritance

It is difficult to disentangle inherited factors from social ones, because related people tend to grow up in similar environments. None the less, there is good evidence from studies of twins and of adopted children that predisposition to both obesity and leanness is at least partially inherited. It has also been shown that the lean children of obese parents eat less than the lean children of lean parents — perhaps compensating for an inherited tendency to get fat.

Congenital syndromes associated with obesity

There are a number of eponymous syndromes characterized by obesity and — usually — hypogonadism and mental subnormality. The commonest is the Prader–Willi syndrome, with a prevalence of 1 : 20 000 births. In the Prader–Willi syndrome hypogonadism and mental subnormality are associated with hypotonia *in utero* (reduced fetal movements) and in infancy (difficulty in sucking). The obesity is caused by gross, and often uncontrollable, overeating.

The Lawrence–Moon–Biedl syndrome combines obesity, hypogonadism, mental subnormality, retinitis pigmentosa and abnormalities of the digits (polydactyly and syndactyly).

Obesity complicating other conditions

Type II diabetes and polycystic ovary syndrome

Both of these are characterized by insulin resistance and a tendency to obesity. In both it is possible that the obesity is the cause of the insulin resistance.

Hypothyroidism

People with hypothyroidism tend to gain weight, but routine screening for hypothyroidism in simple obesity is not justified. People who have had thyrotoxicosis treated, have been rendered hypothyroid and treated with thyroxine, often complain bitterly of difficulty in controlling their weight — even when their serum T_4 concentration is normal. They sometimes respond to treatment with a combination of T_4 and liothyronine.

Hyperprolactinaemia

Hyperprolactinaemia may also be associated with difficulty in losing weight, but the reason is not known.

Cushing's syndrome

Cushing's syndrome is an extremely rare condition and simple obesity is extremely common. Unfortunately, people with simple obesity may share a lot of the physical and biochemical characteristics of corticosteroid excess. Thus they may have diabetes, hypertension, acne, central adiposity and a buffalo hump. Red stretch marks (striae) are also common in young people who gain weight (or height) rapidly, but they are not as broad as in Cushing's. Twenty-four-hour cortisol excretion is increased in obesity, and may be partially resistant to suppression with dexmethasone.

Drug-induced weight gain

Apart from steroids, the commonest drug reported to cause an increase in weight is the combined oral contraceptive, but the evidence for a specific metabolic defect is wanting. Others include phenothiazines (which interfere with central dopaminergic systems) and cyproheptadine (5-HT antagonist).

Caffeine and nicotine

Caffeine stimulates adrenergic β-receptors and facilitates lipolysis. Nicotine stimulates catecholamine release from the adrenal medulla. People who give up smoking have a tendency to gain weight which lasts for up to 2 years. It is part metabolic and part behavioural, with oral satisfaction being achieved with food instead of cigarettes.

CNS control of feeding

People do not become fat unless they eat. They may have a defect in fat metabolism — congenital or acquired — which makes them liable to obesity, but their weight will not increase unless their intake of calories exceeds requirements. The neurochemical mechanisms controlling hunger, appetite, satiety and anorexia are not understood. However, animal studies and observations in humans suggest that the ventromedial nucleus (VMN) of the hypothalamus is involved. Destruction of the VMN is associated with hyperphagia and obesity. Feeding seems to be stimulated by opioid and noradrenergic (α-receptors) nerves, but inhibited by a variety of other neurotransmitter pathways: β-adrenergic, 5-HT, CCK, CRF, TRH, CGRP and insulin.

Recent attention has focused also on neuropeptide Y (NPY), which is present in the hypothalamus and which may stimulate appetite.

It is not clear what role distension of the gastrointestinal tract plays in inducing satiety, or indeed the effect of blood-borne nutrients (glucose and FFAs) on the CNS.

Management of obesity

Doctor–patient relationship

Self-help groups and private slimming clubs probably help more people than doctors and dietitians do. On the other hand, many of the people who seek professional advice have already tried various slimming remedies and have failed. None the less, doctors manage obesity extremely badly and tend to adopt some sort of accusatory role: 'You *must* be eating too much, otherwise you wouldn't be fat' or, with even greater insensitivity, 'There were no fat people in Belsen'.

Accusations of insincerity and self-deceit do little for someone with diminished self-esteem who is struggling hard against an unhelpful metabolism.

It is true that many people who turn to the doctor are looking for some external reason for their problem, and the desire to blame it on 'their hormones' may annoy a doctor who thinks (rightly or wrongly) that the basic problem is greed. However, there is probably little to be gained by trying to discover the real cause of the problem. The object of the consultation is to help the person lose weight, and criticism of their motives and lifestyle encourages neither trust nor compliance. It is better to accept claims of previous strict but unsuccessful dieting on face value, because they will be largely true (even though undermined by binges precipitated by frustration). It helps if it is accepted that fat people do have greater difficulty in losing weight than thin people. What the fat person needs is a sensible diet, combined with professional support and reassurance.

Some 20% of people who ask for medical help will lose significant amounts of weight by dieting, but half will regain it all in the next 2 years. Long-term benefit depends on motivation and on the threats posed by underlying conditions such as diabetes or heart disease. There is no point in asking the advice of a dietitian for someone who has lost weight once and regained it. Similarly, there is no point in seeking dietetic help for someone who has been advised once, and who has failed to lose weight at all.

Weight-reducing diets

The basis of dieting is simple: to lose weight by consuming fewer calories than the body requires to maintain it. The ideal is to reduce fat intake because fat has the highest calorie yield per gram, and to reduce refined carbohydrate. The reason for reducing the intake of sugars is that glucose stimulates the formation of both triglyceride and glycogen. When glycogen is stored, it is stored with water causing an increase in weight. High-fat, high-protein, low-carbohydrate diets have a good short-term effect because of the loss of stored water, but cease to work after 1–2 weeks.

Sometimes the advice given by doctors and dietitians seems illogical to the patient. This applies in particular to insistence on eating three meals a day, albeit small ones. This advice is directed towards the avoidance of binge eating, and towards establishing a better pattern of feeding. Drastic diets can cause drastic weight loss, but dietitians argue that the weight will simply be regained if the person goes back to their former lifestyle. They may be right, but many people find it easier to contemplate a short-term drastic solution rather than a fundamental change in the way they live.

Exercise

Human metabolism was evolved in periods when people were considerably more active physically than today. Increased exercise must be beneficial, even though it will have little effect on body weight unless combined with calorie restriction. Moderate attempts to keep fit consume only a few hundred calories each day.

Behaviour modification

Permanent success requires a long-term change in feeding behaviour. This is difficult because eating habits have been learned by the individual over many years, and will be reinforced by the circumstances of their home life. Eating is a crucial part of human intercourse, playing a central part in many communal activities. Celebrations, holidays and relaxation are nearly always associated with eating unusually large meals. Behaviour modification is the name given to strategies which both promote weight loss, and maintain it.

Many strategies are used, including the creation of a series of progressive short-term targets. These targets may relate to calorie intake ('Confine yourself to 1000 kcal day^{-1}'), or to small amounts of weight lost ('Try and lose 2 kg by this time next month'). One objective is to restore self-esteem and thereby encourage the person to continue dieting. The trouble with many fat people is that they have unrealistic long-term aims: they want to be thin, rather than thinner, and become disillusioned when their efforts are not immediately rewarded.

People who are trying to lose weight are often told to stop weighing themselves and to throw away their bathroom scales. This seems an unnecessary rejection of one means of providing short-term feedback. It is not the scales that need discarding, but the frustration felt in the face of slow progress. Scales should be used, but the person should be encouraged to develop realistic short-term objectives.

Appetite-suppressant drugs

Bulking agents

Swallowing a gelatinous mixture before a meal makes the stomach feel full and reduces the inclination to eat. This is the principle behind the use of bulking agents. They do not work very well.

Amphetamine derivatives acting on adrenergic pathways

Diethylpropion preparations work well at suppressing appetite, but are Listed Drugs because of their tendency to cause central stimulation, and to be addictive.

Amphetamine derivatives acting on 5-HT pathways

Fenfluramine is not addictive and works well as an appetite suppressant. It is likely that tolerance does not develop as often as has been suggested. The main problem with fenfluramine is that is does not cure the underlying feeding problem, and weight is regained when the drug is stopped.

Dexfenfluramine is the d-isomer of fenfluramine and has more specific 5-HT-like action. It has been released only recently, and its clinical value has yet to be assessed. It is not recommended to be used for more than 3 months.

Surgery

Bypass surgery

Bypass surgery of the small bowel (jejunoileal bypass) or stomach cause weight loss by inducing malabsorption. There is a high operative mortality (1–5%), and a longer-term risk of liver failure. Diarrhoea is a common symptom in those who survive. Although weight loss is usually successfully attained, the risks are not justified.

Gastric plication

Gastric plication (gastroplasty) involves stapling the stomach so that only a small part is available for swallowed food. It may have a place in management.

Jaw-wiring

Jaw-wiring works by preventing the person opening their mouth to eat. They therefore depend on a fluid diet for essential nutrition. There is an appreciable risk of aspiration/suffocation if they were to have an accident. Weight is often regained when the wires are removed after a year or so. Jaw-wiring may be effective in the short term, but seems a relatively thoughtless (and potentially dangerous) solution to a complex metabolic and behavioural problem.

Cosmetic surgery

Apronectomy and other forms of fat removal are employed, but will have limited long-term benefit if not combined with dietary modification.

All in all, there is little place for surgery in the management of obesity.

ANOREXIA NERVOSA AND BULIMIA

Anorexia nervosa

It is not clear whether anorexia nervosa is primarily a behavioural disorder causing secondary abnormalities of hypothalamic function, or whether it is a hypothalamic disorder which causes the abnormal feeding. It is likely to be the former since it tends to be more common in selected social groups (especially the ambitious, high-achieving female offspring of professional parents), and it can respond well to psychotherapy. An integral feature of the disorder is an abnormal perception of the desirability of thinness. Many of the defects of endocrine and metabolic function can be ascribed to the consequences of malnutrition: amenorrhoea with suppressed gonadotrophins, high GH, abnormal glucose tolerance and hyperlipidaemia. Serum prolactin concentrations are low in anorexia nervosa.

Management is best undertaken in specialized units. Behaviour modification should be linked to psychotherapy. In many cases the disease is self-limiting: the patient has the intelligence and insight to analyse her (or his) behaviour, and circumstances change.

Bulimia

Bulimia is a related feeding disorder characterized by binge eating with vomiting. It is thought to be a learned behavioural disorder.

Chapter 10
Differentiation, Growth and Development

DIFFERENTIATION

Sexual differentiation

The 'sex' of an individual can be defined in one of four ways: chromosomal sex, gonadal sex, phenotypic sex and behavioural sex. Usually they are the same.

Chromosomal sex

The presence of a Y chromosome causes the development of testes, and generally confers maleness. The histocompatibility Y (H–Y) gene on the Y chromosome leads to the expression of the H–Y cell-surface antigen which signals the primitive gonad to differentiate into a testis. This happens irrespective of the number of X chromosomes (e.g. 47XXY, Klinefelter's syndrome) or Y chromosomes (e.g. 47XYY). When there is no Y chromosome, ovaries develop.

Gonadal sex

The germ cells (which give rise to spermatogonia and oogonia, and ultimately to spermatozoa and ova) are ectodermal and come from the wall of the yolk sac (Fig. 10.1). The other cells of the gonad are from the coelomic epithelium on the medial side of the urogenital ridge, and are mesodermal. In the 4th week of

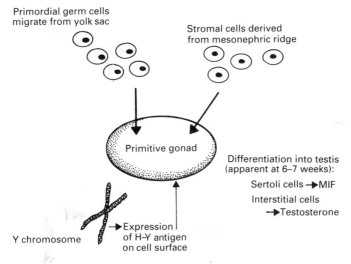

Fig. 10.1. Gonadal differentiation of males. MIF, Mullerian inhibitory factor — also called antimullerian hormone (AMH).

embryological development the ectodermal germ cells migrate to the mesodermal gonadal ridges. The first sign of sexual dimorphism is found in the 6th and 7th weeks when the primordial Sertoli cells (derived from coelomic epithelium, and the equivalent of the granulosa cells of the ovary) of males aggregate into cords. The ovary remains relatively undifferentiated until about the 5th month of gestation, when the primitive granulosa cells become arranged around the dividing oocytes to form primordial follicles.

A testis can develop in the apparent absence of a Y chromosome, but it is extremely rare. While some such cases of 46XX men (estimated prevalence 1 in 20 000 male births) may be mosaics and have undetected Y chromosomes, it is thought that the majority have an aberrant H–Y gene on an X chromosome.

True hermaphroditism is the name given to the association of both ovarian and testicular tissue in the same individual. The person may have either two mixed ovotestes, or have one testis and one ovary (sometimes with hemidifferentiation of the internal and external genitalia as well). It may be caused by mosaicism, or by the presence of H–Y-determining tissue on X chromosomes. Over 60% are 46XX, 10% are 46XY, and the remainder are mosaics.

Phenotypic sex

In mammals the induced phenotype is male. In other words, a castrated embryo will develop into a female.

Internal genitalia

The female phenotype is characterized by the persistence of the Mullerian ducts (Fig. 10.2). These form the Fallopian tubes and uterus. The primitive Wolffian ducts do not develop. In males the Mullerian ducts regress in response to the secretion of Mullerian inhibitory factor (MIF). This is a dimeric glycoprotein (molecular weight 140 000 Da) which is secreted by the Sertoli cells. At the same time, development of the Wolffian duct into the internal genitalia (the epididymes, vasa deferentia, seminal vesicles and prostate) occurs. This is triggered by the secretion of androgens. The testes secrete testosterone from about the 6th week of gestation (Fig. 10.3).

External genitalia

The development of the external genitalia in males is also dependent on androgens, in particular on dihydrotestosterone (DHT), which is derived from testosterone in target tissues. The formation of DHT is not necessary for the differentiation of internal genitalia. Thus individuals who do not produce DHT (see Syndromes of androgen resistance, p. 178) have normal internal genitalia (induced by testosterone), but feminized external genitalia (because of lack of DHT).

Other aspects of physical development, including breast structure, are identical in males and females until the onset of puberty (Fig. 10.4).

Behavioural sex

There is some evidence that it is exposure of the fetal brain to testosterone (not DHT) which determines male-type sexual behaviour in most individuals. As DHT is not involved, boys with Reifenstein's syndrome (reduced conversion of

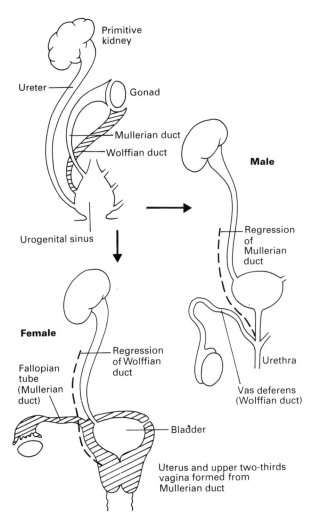

Fig. 10.2. Differentiation of internal genitalia.

testosterone to DHT) have partial feminization of the external genitalia, but a sexual orientation which is male.

Sexual behaviour in humans is also determined by social and psychological factors, and these presumably condition the transient homosexuality which is common in adolescence. There is no known endocrine basis for homosexual behaviour in either men or women. Nor is there generally any endocrinological difference between people who are more or less sexually active.

None the less excessive circulating androgens may exaggerate libido in women, and gross deficiency of gonadal steroids will reduce libido in either sex. Men with hypogonadism who are treated with intermittent injections of testosterone may have exaggerated libido for several days after an injection, but it is reduced by the time the next injection is due.

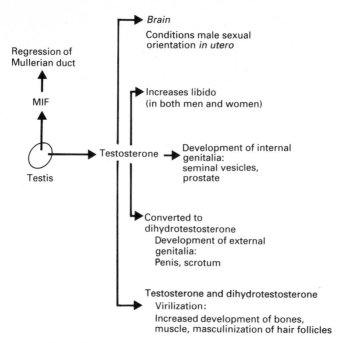

Fig. 10.3. Phenotypic male sex. MIF, Mullerian inhibitory factor.

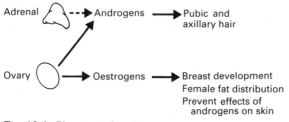

Fig. 10.4. Phenotypic female sex.

Abnormalities of sexual development

Traditional classification

True hermaphroditism

The presence of both ovarian and testicular tissue in the same person.

Male pseudohermaphroditism

Chromosomal sex is male and testes are present, but there is variable feminization of the internal and external genitalia.

Female pseudohermaphroditism

Chromosomal sex is female and ovaries are present, but there is variable masculinization of the internal and external genitalia.

Table 10.1. Effect of hormones on the differentiation of external genitalia

---

Testosterone from the Leydig cells of the fetal testis causes development of the internal genitalia (Wolffian duct derivatives)

MIF (AMH) from the Sertoli cells causes regression of the Mullerian duct.

Testosterone is converted to DHT by the enzyme 5α-reductase, and DHT causes the development of external genitalia

---

Male and female pseudohermaphroditism are caused by endocrine abnormalities, because it is hormones that determine the differentiation of the non-gonadal genitalia (Table 10.1). The term 'hermaphroditism' is not ideal, however, because of the perorative stigma attached to it. An alternative classification for intersex states follows.

Alternative classification

Gross chromosomal abnormalities
With conflict between chromosomal sex and gonadal sex:
1 Both testes and ovaries present.
2 46XX male.
3 46XY female.
4 Many variants and mosaics.
With no conflict between chromosomal sex and gonadal sex: individuals with a Y chromosome have testes and those without have ovaries, but phenotypic sex is abnormal.

47XXY: Klinefelter's syndrome
Individuals are male but with variable degrees of primary hypogonadism. They are nearly always infertile because of abnormal development of the seminiferous tubules, but some have normal Leydig cells with adequate testosterone secretion and are well virilized. If the Leydig cells are defective as well as the seminiferous tubules, the individual will be tall (eunuchoidal) with hypogonadal features and gynaecomastia. The testes are usually small (5–6 ml) and firm. Testosterone concentration in the blood may be normal or low. Serum follicle-stimulating hormone (FSH) is high. Intellectual achievement may be slightly reduced.

47XYY syndrome (and variants)
This includes phenotypic males who are not hypogonadal, but who were at one time said to have a higher prevalence of mental subnormality associated with violent tendencies. This is wrong: 47XYY seems to be a variant compatible with normal life development and behaviour.

46XO (and variants): Turner's syndrome
The ovaries undergo normal early differentiation but exaggerated oocyte depletion, and fibrosis is apparent from the 14th to the 16th weeks of gestation. In the

adult the ovary is usually represented by a mere streak of fibrous tissue. This is not always the case, however, and some women with Turner's syndrome have occasional periods. Breast development is poor (low oestrogens); external genitalia are normal but prepubertal prior to oestrogen replacement therapy.

Affected women may have other somatic features: small stature, web neck (pterygiocollis), wide carrying angle (cubitus valgus), congenital cardiac malformations, low-set ears, shield-shaped chest (wide-spaced nipples) and slanting eyes.

Male Turner's syndrome
Affected males are 46XY, but have some of the features of female Turner's syndrome. They may have normal testes or be hypogonadal.

No gross chromosomal abnormalities

Syndromes of androgen excess (female pseudohermaphroditism)
If androgens circulate in excessive concentrations in a female fetus, she will develop virilization of the external genitalia. This is nearly always the result of congenital adrenal hyperplasia (CAH). Other known causes are androgen-secreting tumours in the mother, or iatrogenic (exposure of the mother to androgens while she is pregnant). Apart from CAH, most cases are unexplained.

Syndromes of androgen resistance (male pseudohermaphroditism)
In secondary sexual tissues testosterone is converted to DHT by the cytoplasmic enzyme 5α-reductase. There is a cytosolic receptor for both testosterone and DHT. DHT is transported to the nucleus to induce DNA replication.

In syndromes of androgen resistance, testosterone and/or DHT are ineffective, or only partially effective. There are three main reasons:
1 Defect in the cytosolic receptor.
2 Post-receptor defect.
3 5α-reductase deficiency.

Receptor and post-receptor testosterone resistance
Receptor and post-receptor defects are clinically indistinguishable. The degree of severity of the defect determines the clinical presentation. More severe defects are phenotypically more female; milder ones are more virilized.
1 *Female phenotype — testicular feminization:* as neither testosterone nor DHT are active, the person has no male internal genitalia (the Wolffian system needs testosterone), but no female genitalia either (MIF is normal). Externally the person develops a normal female phenotype except for absent body hair and a short blind vagina (no Mullerian component, see Fig. 10.2). Sexual orientation is female, because testosterone is ineffective on the developing brain. Testicular feminization may be complete or partial.
2 *Male phenotype — Reifenstein's syndrome:* the external genitalia are more male, and the children are raised as boys. As adults they have a male sexual orientation. The external genitalia are variably maldeveloped — small penis, hypospadias. They have gynaecomastia, but body form is otherwise male.

3 *Male phenotype — 5α-reductase deficiency*
The testosterone is active (normal Wolffian structures, internal genitalia), but there is deficient DHT. This results in defective formation of the external genitalia, but the individuals are male in every other way.

Principles of management of intersex states

Management will usually be determined in specialized centres, but the principles are:
1 Ensure that the gender assignment is the most appropriate for that individual.
2 Treat deficiency of sex hormones with replacement therapy to ensure, when appropriate, as much secondary sexual development as possible, and to prevent osteoporosis in later life.
3 Plastic surgery to remedy abnormal external genitalia.
4 Remove any abnormal testicular tissue because of the very high risk of neoplasia. The risk is mainly confined to those with Y chromosomes. The commonest tumours (gonadoblastomas) are benign.
5 Genetic counselling.

Other abnormalities of intrauterine development

Hypospadias
Formation of the penis involves the ventral fusion of the genital swellings (primitive labia majora). This can be incomplete, with the urethral meatus opening proximal to the glans.

Micropenis
Some boys have a very small penis — < 2.5 cm stretched length. This may reflect hypopituitarism or primary hypogonadism with reduced fetal testosterone production, or it may reflect a partial defect in DHT production or action (see Syndromes of androgen resistance, p. 178). Hypopituitarism may also cause neonatal hypoglycaemia (due to glucocorticoid deficiency) and hypothyroidism. Hypopituitary babies are not small, however, because intrauterine growth depends more on the production of IGF_2 in fetal tissues than on the pituitary secretion of growth hormone (GH).

Cryptorchidism: incomplete and maldescent of the testis
The testes normally migrate to the scrotum through the inguinal canal during the 7th intrauterine month. The mechanism is not known but probably depends on the baby's luteinizing hormone (LH) as well as on placental human chorionic gonadotrophin (hCG). Cryptorchidism is present in approximately 3% of those delivered at term, but is more common in premature babies. It must be distinguished from abnormally retractile (in response to cold or anxiety) testes. If cryptorchid testes are to descend spontaneously later, it is nearly always within the first few months of life. Eighty per cent of cryptorchid testes are capable of normal function. The prevalence by school age is less than 1%.

Maldescent of the testes (ectopic testes) is much less common. Anorchia is very rare indeed (100 times less common than cryptorchidism). The testes are intact in early intrauterine life, but atrophy in a way similar to the ovaries in Turner's syndrome.

The cause of cryptorchidism is not known, although it is possible that testes that do not descend properly are congenitally abnormal, and this may explain the high incidence of neoplasia.

Cryptorchid testes are hypoplastic, but it is not possible to tell whether this is the cause or the consequence of maldescent. Testes which remain within, or close to, the abdominal cavity do not develop normally because it is too warm. They carry a 10-fold risk of neoplasm formation in adulthood, even if surgically repositioned in the scrotum. It follows that testes which are not functioning (the person is hypogonadal, and requires androgen replacement therapy as an adult) should be removed.

Treatment

Surgical repositioning (orchidopexy) is usually attempted at 3–4 years of age. When the defect is less marked (high scrotal position), it may respond to treatment with hCG (500–4000 U i.m. two to three times weekly for 3–6 weeks). If the response is good, it is likely that descent will be completed spontaneously as the child goes through puberty. Endocrine treatment may also improve the success of surgery. The administration of gonadotrophin-releasing hormone (GnRH) by intranasal spray has also been shown to work.

GROWTH AND DEVELOPMENT

Growth

Growth hormone, growth factors and gonadal steroids

Growth involves the division and differentiation of all cells. It requires GH as well as a range of other hormones and growth factors, particularly insulin and insulin-like growth factors (IGF_1 and IGF_2).

In the fetus most growth seems to depend on IGF_2 formed in the tissues, and is independent of GH: GH-deficient children are not small at birth, and this is not because of the effect of the mother's GH because GH does not cross the placenta. Growth becomes GH-dependent after birth, and is most rapid in the first 2 years of life (Fig. 10.5). GH stimulates the formation of IGF_1 and IGF_2 in the liver as well as in peripheral tissues (see Fig. 2.7). IGF_1 concentrations rise slowly through childhood, while IGF_2 concentrations fall. IGF_1 correlates best with body size, and IGF_2 correlates with height velocity (Fig. 10.6).

In the cartilage of the epiphyses, at the growing ends of long bones, stem cells proliferate and differentiate into bone cells under the influence of IGFs. This area is called the growth plate (Fig. 10.7). When there is insufficient calcium or vitamin D available, the growth plate is widened because the cells are unable to calcify the newly formed woven bone. This happens in rickets.

Gonadal steroids stimulate the secretion of GH by the pituitary, and this is the reason for the growth spurt which coincides with gonadal development in puberty. However, gonadal steroids also terminate growth: they reduce the blood supply to

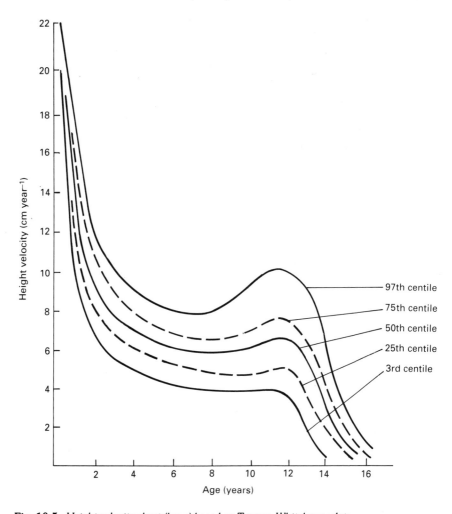

Fig. 10.5. Height velocity chart (boys) based on Tanner–Whitehouse data.

the growth plate, and eventually the epiphyses fuse with the metaphysis (Fig. 10.7).

Growth in childhood

Linear growth (height velocity) falls from 20 cm per year at birth to 10 cm per year at age 2. It then declines progessively each year to about 5 cm per year immediately before the puberty growth spurt (see Fig. 10.5). Most of this growth is dependent on GH secretion and on the IGFs (particularly IGF_1), which it induces, even though GH-deficient children do grow a little (basal growth). Growth hormone is secreted mainly in bursts, during Stage IV sleep. As the gonads start to develop, increasing serum concentrations of sex steroids stimulate the pituitary to secrete more frequent and bigger bursts of GH (Fig. 10.8).

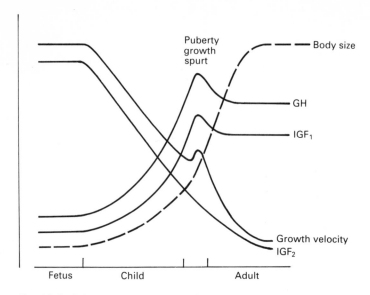

Fig. 10.6. Schematic representation of changes in growth hormone (GH) and insulin-like growth factors (IGFs) with increasing age.

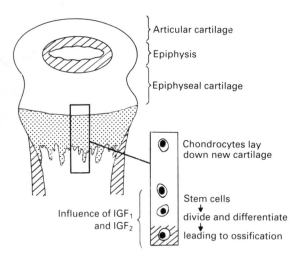

Fig. 10.7. Diagrammatic representation of the growing end of a long bone.

Small stature in childhood

Of the 30 per 1000 children whose height falls below the 3rd centile, only one or two will have treatable organic disease. Up to 30% of cases of small stature can be attributed to social deprivation; GH deficiency affects only one child in 4000. None the less, those who lie below the 3rd centile should be considered for specialist referral.

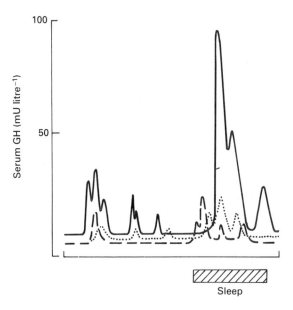

Fig. 10.8. Increase in serum GH through puberty. Shown are 24 hour profiles of serum GH concentration in childhood (– – –), early puberty (· · ·), and late puberty (——).

Causes of small stature

Familial or constitutional
If the parents are small, it usually indicates an inherited trait — although it should be remembered that the parents might be small because they suffered social deprivation when growing, and their children might be suffering similarly. Children with other congenital abnormalities may be constitutionally small. Rarely, a short girl whose mother is also short, with bowed legs, may be found to have vitamin D-resistant rickets — hypophosphataemia.

Social and emotional deprivation
Adverse factors in the environment result in disordered sleep, with abnormal sleep-related GH secretion.

Systemic disease
Children with systemic disease may be small. The disease may or may not be previously recognized: coeliac disease, poorly controlled diabetes, hypothyroidism or treated arthropathies such as juvenile rheumatoid arthritis.

GH deficiency
Idiopathic hypothalamic growth-hormone releasing hormone (GHRH) deficiency is the commonest cause of low GH levels, but children might have structural

disease of the hypothalamus or pituitary, such as craniopharyngioma or pituitary tumour.

Growth hormone resistance (Laron-type dwarfism)

Inherited deficiency of GH receptors is associated with low serum IGF_1 concentrations and short stature. GH levels are high. It is extremely rare.

Clinical

History-taking should be directed at defining details of the child's developmental, social and family circumstances. Examination should exclude obvious associated organic disease. Socially deprived children tend to be thin, whereas GH-deficient or hypothyroid children tend to be plump.

Investigations

A blood sample should be taken after exercise (vigorous exercise may produce a peak in serum cortisol and GH secretion after a delay of 15 minutes) to exclude systemic disease, and chromosomal abnormalities (Turner's syndrome is a relatively common disorder in girls). Full blood count, erythrocyte sedimentation rate (ESR), urea and electrolytes, thyroid function tests (TFTs), GH and cortisol should be measured, as well as IGF_1 (if available). Urine should be checked to exclude diabetes insipidus (low osmolality), diabetes mellitus and occult infection. X-rays should be taken of the skull (to exclude obvious intracranial disease), and hand and wrist (for bone age).

Bone age

The appearance and maturation of the epiphyses (bone age) is essential for the prediction of final height. If bone age is delayed (beyond chronological age), there is potential for catch-up growth (Fig. 10.9). Children with constitutional small stature have no delay in bone age.

Height record

This should only be done in specialized centres. Height is measured each 3–6 months using a Harpenden stadiometer. Actual height is plotted on Tanner charts, and growth velocity calculated. Height which is inexplicably below the 3rd centile, and height velocity below the 25th centile are usually indications for detailed assessment of GH reserve — provided that other problems have been excluded, and provided the result of the earlier GH sample was < 15 mU litre^{-1}.

Biochemical assessment of GH reserve

A number of different tests are used to establish that GH reserve is normal:

1 Insulin stress test — 0.05–0.1 U kg^{-1}. It induces hypoglycaemia, which is potentially dangerous.
2 Oral clonidine — 0.15 mg m^{-2}. Hypotension occurs occasionally.
3 Arginine i.v. — 0.5 g kg^{-1} (max. 40 g) infused over 30 min. This test can be combined with an insulin stress test.
4 Glucagon i.m. — 30–100 µg kg^{-1} s.c. or i.m. Makes children sick.

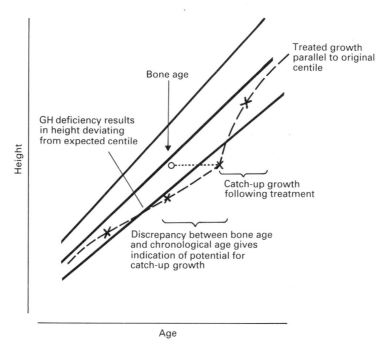

Fig. 10.9. Use of bone age to estimate potential for catch-up growth.

5 Documentation of peak GH during Stage IV sleep. Good — especially for the very young, but inconvenient if EEG monitoring is used.

6 Overnight or 24-hour serum GH profile, with samples taken every 20 minutes.

7 GHRH administration helps define pituitary GH reserve but does not help determine the need for GH treatment.

The object of all tests is to demonstrate that serum GH can reach a peak of over 15 mU litre^{-1}. If it does, GH therapy is not indicated. None of the tests are completely reliable: normal children may not produce a normal peak > 15 mU litre^{-1}. They are more likely to if they are given sex steroids before the test is done. Girls should be given 100 µg ethinyloestradiol orally for 3 days. Boys can be treated either with ethinyloestradiol, or with a single i.m. injection of 100 mg testosterone esters (Sustanon or Primoteston) 3 days before the test. Sex steroid priming should not be done if bone age is < 10 years.

Treatment

Treatment of GH deficiency involves twice- or thrice-weekly injections s.c. or i.m. of recombinant human GH (12–15 U week^{-1} or 0.5 U kg^{-1} week^{-1}). Height velocities of up to 10 cm year^{-1} can be achieved in children who respond, but not all do. Sometimes gonadal steroids (boys — 100 mg testosterone month^{-1}; girls — 5–10 µg ethinyloestradiol daily) are given to enhance the response to GH, but there is a risk of causing early epiphyseal fusion and stunting final adult height, because gonadal steroids may hasten epiphyseal closure.

GH for constitutional short stature

There is no evidence that GH benefits children who are short for reasons other than GH deficiency.

GH and Creutzfeld–Jakob disease

The treatment of GH deficiency before 1985 involved the use of GH purified from human pituitary glands taken at post-mortem. By 1990 it was apparent that a small but significant number (eight in the UK) of people treated in this way had developed CJD: progressive destruction of the cerebral cortex leading over several years to dementia and death — the result of slow virus infection. It is not possible to define whether or not others who were treated will later develop CJD. CJD is untreatable.

Since 1985 all GH has been produced by recombinant DNA technology and there is no risk of slow virus infection.

Tall stature

Tall children are usually constitutionally tall. However, some conditions need to be considered.

Congenital adrenal hyperplasias

The increased secretion of adrenal androgens results in increased GH secretion. A growth spurt similar to the one which occurs during normal puberty commences at the age of 3 or 4 years. In infancy the child is very much taller (and muscular) than normal, but final height is stunted because of premature fusion of the epiphyses (see pp. 92–6).

Precocious puberty

If a child goes into early puberty there will be a puberty growth spurt.

Thyrotoxicosis

Thyroid hormones stimulate GH secretion and this can cause abnormal tallness, especially when thyrotoxicosis occurs in the teenage years.

Hypogonadism

If an otherwise normal person has congenital hypogonadism (e.g. due to isolated GnRH deficiency), they will be tall with eunuchoid proportions. The absence of sex steroids causes delayed fusion of the epiphyses, and linear growth stimulated by GH continues for longer than it normally would. The long bones are affected more than the axial skeleton. Span normally equals height, but eunuchoid people have a span greater than 2 cm more than height (see Fig. 2.12).

GH-secreting pituitary tumour

Older children with GH-secreting tumours become progressively tall. If the tumour is a large one and gonadotrophin secretion is compromised, gonadal maturation will not occur, sex steroid levels will be low and the epiphyses will not fuse. The child becomes a giant.

Puberty

Puberty refers to the process of sexual maturation — from childhood to adulthood. It requires complex integration between the pineal, pituitary, adrenals and gonads, and involves growth and maturation of the whole body. The onset of menstruation (menarche) is often regarded loosely as the time of puberty in girls, but it is better to regard the menarche as merely one stage — neither the first nor the last — of a process which takes several years.

The first change occurs at about the age of 6–8 years, and is a maturation of the adrenal enzymes which control steroidogenesis. The result is an increased secretion of adrenal androgens. Over the next 4 or 5 years these stimulate the development of pubic and axillary hair, although most hair growth results from the later secretion of androgens by the ovaries and testes.

During childhood the hypothalamus and pituitary are abnormally sensitive to the negative feedback effect of circulating steroids. When this sensitivity is reduced — because of a fall in melatonin production by the pineal — the secretion of LH and FSH increases, with pulses of increased size and frequency, especially during sleep. LH stimulates testicular development in boys and serum testosterone rises. FSH stimulates early maturation of ovarian follicles, with secretion of both androgens and oestrogens.

Rising gonadal steroid levels stimulate the pituitary to secrete larger pulses of GH. This causes increased IGF production by the liver, and the child enters the puberty growth spurt. Girls start to grow at an earlier age than boys. Boys are therefore taller at the onset of the puberty growth spurt and this may explain why their final adult height is greater.

The staging of growth and sexual development in Caucasian children in England in the 1960s was documented by Tanner and Whitehouse, and the Tanner charts are now used as standards for clinical practice. These charts refer to increases in height, weight, pubic hair, penis and scrotum and breasts (Table 10.2).

Gonadal steroids both initiate the growth spurt and also terminate it. Testosterone (and, probably, oestradiol) enhances GH secretion, but also eventually causes fusion of the epiphyseal plates by altering their blood supply.

Spermatogenesis occurs from a very early stage of the maturation process in boys — often long before the other signs of sexual maturity are marked. Genital development occurs relatively early, but full muscular development and hair growth are slowly progressive until the age of 20 and beyond. Hair follicles are relatively slow to respond to the increasing androgens, and hairs on the chest are often not maximal until the mid-20s. Approximately 50% of boys develop breast enlargement in puberty, probably due to the conversion of testosterone to oestrogens in peripheral tissues.

Delayed puberty

Ninety-seven per cent of children enter puberty by the age of 14, and will go on to full maturation over the succeeding 4–5 years. However, those who reach 14 and have no sign of puberty should be referred for assessment — even though they are very unlikely to have any specific endocrine abnormality. They may

Table 10.2. Tanner staging

Boys: genital development
Stage 1	Pre-adolescent — same as in early childhood
Stage 2	Enlargement of testes. Scrotum enlarges, becomes redder, and rougher in texture
Stage 3	Penis lengthens. Testes and scrotum enlarge further
Stage 4	Penis broader, development of glans. Scrotum darkens
Stage 5	Adult

Girls: breast development
Stage 1	Pre-adolescent: elevation of papilla only
Stage 2	Breast bud: small mound. Areola enlarges
Stage 3	Further enlargement but no separation of contours of papilla and areola from the breast
Stage 4	Elevation of areola and papilla above curve of breast
Stage 5	Mature: papilla elevated but areola flattens into breast contour

Both sexes: pubic hair
Stage 1	Pre-adolescent
Stage 2	Sparse growth of darker, longer hairs on labia or at base of penis
Stage 3	Darker, thicker and more curly, covering junction of pubes
Stage 4	Adult in type but not as extensive
Stage 5	Adult in type, spreading up linea alba and onto medial aspect of thighs — especially in men

---

have idiopathic delay (i.e. the extreme end of the normal spectrum). Alternatively, they may have delay caused by systemic disease or by psychosocial problems.

It is a mistake, however, to underestimate the distress caused by the problem and treatment with sex hormones is often indicated, even in the absence of a specific underlying hormone problem.

Causes

There are both non-endocrine causes and endocrine causes; the endocrine causes are very uncommon.

Non-endocrine causes
1 Social deprivation.
2 Inherited or constitutional.
3 Non-endocrine systemic disease: diabetes, inflammatory bowel disease, Still's disease, asthma, malabsorption.
4 Treatment of systemic disease, especially with glucocorticoids.

Endocrine causes
1 Hypothalamic or pituitary disease causing both GH deficiency and gonadotrophin deficiency.

Table 10.3. Investigation of delayed puberty

Full blood count, ESR, urea and electrolytes, glucose
X-ray hand for bone age
Prolactin, TFTs
Testosterone (boys)
Ovarian ultrasound (girls)
Karyotype if significant gonadal disease is suspected
Tests of GH and ACTH reserve if pituitary disease is suspected

2 Hypothyroidism: hypothyroid children may or may not be otherwise obviously myxoedematous, but tend to be overweight.

Assessment

The detailed assessment is described in the investigation of small stature (Table 10.3). If there are definite signs of early puberty on examination, both child and parent may be content to be reassured that changes are imminent. This is especially true in boys if the testosterone is found to be in or near the adult reference range. Ovarian ultrasound (repeated if necessary) in girls may show follicular activity. There is no need for such children to be followed more frequently than 6-monthly. Once it is clear that development is proceeding, the child/young person should be discharged, to minimize any self-consciousness and feeling of being 'abnormal'.

Dynamic tests

Neither the GnRH test nor the clomiphene test is of diagnostic value in the younger teenager with delayed puberty. Stimulation of the testes with hCG (hCG stimulation test: 500 U i.m. daily for 3 days with measurement of testosterone on days 0,3 and 5) will help exclude primary disease of the testes in boys.

Isolated GnRH deficiency and Kallman's syndrome can be very difficult to diagnose in early teenage. It may only become obvious when a trial of treatment fails to trigger normal development.

Treatment (irrespective of cause)

In some cases the child/young person is obviously very disadvantaged and/or embarrassed, and it is not sufficient to reassure and wait — even though it is believed that normal development will take place eventually. Boys can be treated with a short course of either hCG to stimulate their own testes (500–1500 U i.m. two or three times a week for 6 weeks) or testosterone (Sustanon or Primoteston 100 mg i.m. monthly for 3 months). It is probably better to opt for testosterone because it means fewer injections. GnRH can be given by continuous pulsatile infusion but it is not widely used. An alternative approach in boys is to give low doses of anabolic steroids, oxandrolone (1.25 mg daily) or fluoxymesterone, for 3 months. Anabolic steroids in low doses will stimulate GH release and initiate a growth spurt, but will not cause premature fusion of the epiphyses.

It is more usual to withhold treatment in girls with constitutional delay, but breast development and growth can be stimulated with low doses of ethinyl oestradiol (1 µg daily for 6 months, 5 µg for 6 months, 10 µg for 6 months). There is no evidence that this approach delays or modifies final development in any way, but the onset of some sign of development can be a great boost to the patient.

If the delay is not constitutional, the child needs long-term therapy with sex steroids. Boys should be given Sustanon or Primoteston 100 mg each 4 weeks (increasing to 250 mg each 2–4 weeks in adulthood). Adults can also be treated with 6-monthly testosterone implants. Transdermal administration of testosterone by skin patches may soon be available. If the person wishes to father children, they require treatment with hCG and FSH (see Fig. 2.13).

Girls should be treated long-term with a cyclical regimen including a progestogen. Mercilon is a convenient oral contraceptive preparation containing only 20 µg ethinyl oestradiol. Ovulation can be induced with hCG and FSH when fertility becomes a consideration — provided the ovaries are capable of responding.

Delayed puberty in the older teenager

Older teenagers present with either delayed puberty and small stature, or delayed puberty and normal or tall stature. Those with delayed puberty and small stature usually have constitutional delay; those who are taller are often hypogonadal — hypothalamic GnRH deficiency or pituitary disease.

Clinical examination may reveal signs of established syndromes, such as Turner's syndrome (46XO) or Klinefelter's (47XXY). An absent sense of smell or colour blindness suggests Kallman's syndrome (where these are associated with GnRH deficiency).

Someone who is hypogonadal in late teenage, and yet who has normal GH secretion, will be eunuchoid. A hypogonadal male may have gynaecomastia due to androgen deficiency.

Biochemical assessment

Diagnosis of GnRH deficiency is sometimes easier in older teenagers. The classic finding is that the person has a good rise in serum LH and FSH in the 60 minutes following the i.v. injection of GnRH, but no rise in LH and FSH in the clomiphene test (3 mg kg^{-1} clomiphene orally for 10 days). It is not completely diagnostic, however, because this pattern can also be found in older teenagers with idiopathic delay.

Other tests

1   LH and FSH will be high if there is primary gonadal failure (e.g. dysgenesis, Klinefelter's, Turner's or cryptorchidism).
2   Prolactin may be high if the hypogonadism is caused by a prolactinoma or other pituitary disease.
3   TFTs: hypothyroidism can cause reversible hypogonadism.
4   Karyotype may reveal chromosomal abnormalities.
5   Testosterone in males; ovarian ultrasound in girls.

Precocious puberty

When the gonads develop prematurely (i.e. earlier than 2 times SD before the mean — about 8 years in girls, 9.5 years in boys), the condition is called precocious puberty. As the gonads develop, the child develops the secondary sexual characteristics of an adult. When the secondary sexual characteristics develop without the gonads, the condition is called precocious pseudopuberty. In fact, this only ever happens in untreated CAH.

Causes

Precocious puberty in girls is nearly always idiopathic. Precocious puberty in boys is often caused by significant intracranial disease (Table 10.4).

Central precocious puberty

True precocious puberty is also called central precocious puberty — 90% of cases occur in girls. They are usually idiopathic, although small hypothalamic hamartomata may sometimes be seen on CT scan. These hamartomata are of no pathological significance and do not affect management.

McCune–Albright syndrome

McCune and Albright were the first authors of papers published separately in 1937, describing this rare condition. It affects girls, and they suffer precocious puberty (apparently caused by autonomous ovarian steriod secretion — i.e. independent of gonadotrophins), patchy ('geographical') skin pigmentation, and polyostotic fibrous dysplasia. The last of these abnormalities can cause the greatest disability, with recurrent painless fractures healing with bony deformity. However, the disease is relatively benign and the bone manifestations cease in adulthood. It is extremely rare.

Table 10.4. Organic causes of precocious puberty

Organic brain syndromes
These can trigger abnormally early secretion of LH and FSH:
  Hydrocephalus
  Tumours: neoplasia, especially pinealomas, von Recklinghausen's disease
  Conditions associated with mental subnormality, e.g. Down's syndrome
  Space-occupying lesions in the region of the tuber cinereum

Tumours secreting hCG
These stimulate the testes directly, leaving the hypothalamus and pituitary suppressed
  Intracranial teratomas
  Other teratomas
  Hepatomas

Primary gonadal: McCune–Albright syndrome

Clinical

The consequences of precocious puberty are physical and psychosocial. The physical consequences are that the child enters an abnormally early puberty growth spurt, but also stops growing equally early, so that final adult height is stunted. The psychosocial consequences result from the abnormal interest taken in the child's development, both by adults and by other children. This results in a sense of isolation and embarrassment. These may be exacerbated by unnatural social and psychological expectations being made of a child whose intellectual development does not keep pace with its physical development. The child may be at increased risk of sexual abuse.

Assessment

The assessment of precocious puberty is directed at:

1 Establishing the diagnosis by clinical examination, and by testosterone assay in boys, assay of oestradiol/progesterone and ovarian ultrasound in girls.

2 Demonstrating that the problem is central (i.e. LH- and FSH-dependent) by GnRH test: adult responses of LH and FSH to the i.v. injection of 100 µg GnRH.

3 Excluding significant intracranial disease — CT scan.

4 Assessing anticipated final adult height: bone age — precocious puberty advances bone age, with premature closure of the epiphyses.

Treatment

In idiopathic precocious puberty it is sometimes enough to exclude underlying disease and to leave the child untreated. However, it is more usual to try to suppress gonadotrophin secretion and gonadal function using progestogens. The objective is partly to allow the child to develop at the same time as their peers, but more importantly, to arrest accelerated bone maturation. If given early enough, it improves the final height prognosis.

Cyproterone acetate is a progestogen which is also a powerful antiandrogen. It suppresses androgen synthesis and blocks their action on target cells. As a progestogen it also suppresses gonadotrophin secretion. It is effective in idiopathic precocious puberty in doses of 25–100 mg daily. Suppression of gonadotrophin secretion can also be achieved with the progestogen medroxy-progesterone acetate.

Intranasal administration of GnRH analogues (e.g. buserelin) is also effective and may become the treatment of choice for central precocious puberty. Although they are GnRH-like, they are so potent that they cause down-regulation of the pituitary with a paradoxical reduction in LH and FSH secretion.

Chapter 11
Male Sexual Function — Andrology

THE TESTIS

The testis is the major source of testosterone. It is also the site of spermatogenesis.

Development

The germ cells are derived from the yolk-sac wall and are ectodermal. They migrate in the 4th week of gestation to the gonadal ridge, which is mesodermal. The start of differentiation of the testis into seminiferous tubules and interstitium is apparent by the 7th week, and the testes normally move through the inguinal canal into the scrotum in the 7th month. The interstitial (Leydig) cells are prominent through intrauterine life as a result of stimulation by placental human chorionic gonadotrophin (hCG): hCG has actions similar to luteinizing hormone (LH). At the time of birth, serum levels of testosterone in boys are of the same order as in adult men, but they fall rapidly as the interstitial cells regress in the absence of hCG.

Anatomy

The normal adult testis is 20–25 ml in volume and encapsulated by the tunica albuginea — a tough fibrous layer containing scattered myoepithelial (contractile) cells. The interstitial cells are packed together, together with vessels and prominent lymphatics, between the seminiferous tubules. The tubules are also lined by a layer of contractile myoepithelial cells. Within the tubules there are two main types of cells — germ cells, lining the basement membrane as spermatogonia, but evolving into spermatocytes, spermatids and spermatozoa towards the centre of the tubular lumen — and Sertoli cells. Sertoli (sustentacular, supporting) cells retain very close anatomical and functional contact with the developing spermatozoa (Fig. 11.1). They both secrete, and have receptors for, a large number of hormones and locally acting growth factors.

Hormonal control of the testis

LH stimulates the interstitial cells to secrete testosterone, while follicle-stimulating hormone (FSH) and testosterone together stimulate the seminiferous tubules to produce spermatozoa. Testosterone reduces the secretion of LH by a negative feedback effect on the pituitary (and/or hypothalamus). Negative feedback of FSH secretion is mediated by inhibin, a two-chain polypeptide hormone released from the Sertoli cells during the process of spermatogenesis. They also secrete activin, which is a dimer of inhibin, and which has opposite actions on the pituitary — it stimulates FSH secretion. Individuals with interstitial cell failure and primary hypogonadism causing low concentrations of testosterone will have high

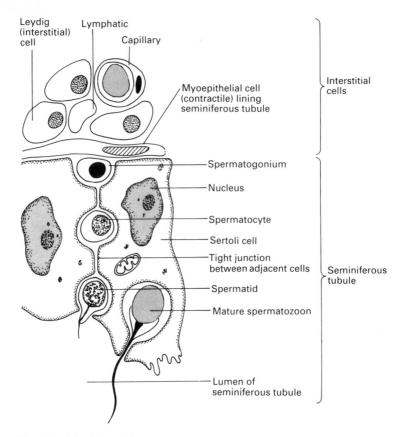

Fig. 11.1. Structure of the testis.

levels of LH, while those with impaired spermatogenesis will have high FSH levels (Fig. 11.2).

Maturity and ageing

During childhood the testes enlarge slowly but testosterone concentrations remain low. At the onset of puberty, increasing release of the gonadotrophins LH and FSH causes hypertrophy of the interstitial cells, and final maturation of the seminiferous tubules follows. The onset of spermatogenesis occurs early in puberty, long before the boy has developed full secondary sexual characteristics. Increasing concentrations of testosterone result in maturation of the external genitalia, the development of sex hormone-dependent body hair (facial, pubic, axillary), puberty growth spurt and progressive virilization. The rise in androgens is associated with transient breast enlargement (puberty gynaecomastia), because testosterone is aromatized to form oestrogens.

Some men go through a 'male climacteric' as they grow older — equivalent to the menopause. There is progressive primary gonadal failure, with falling testosterone concentrations and rising LH and FSH. Most men do not: testosterone and gonadotrophin levels remain unchanged until old age.

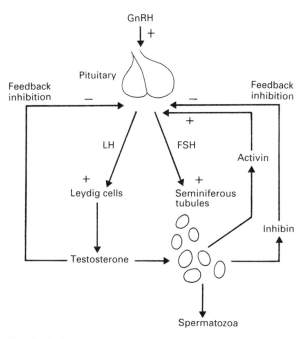

Fig. 11.2. Hormonal control of the testis.

ERECTION AND IMPOTENCE

Erections are not dependent on hormones: castrated males can have erections, and boys have erections right through childhood, when serum testosterone levels are very low. None the less, people think that sex is all to do with hormones, and endocrinologists are often asked for help, and that is why the subject is discussed here.

Physiology of erection

In order to obtain an erection, a man must have a penis which is of the right size and shape. The internal pudendal arteries must be capable of transmitting up to 100 ml min^{-1} of arterial blood. The medium-sized arteries and arterioles of the penis must, together with the corpora cavernosa, be capable of distributing blood appropriately. There must be an intact mechanism for impeding venous drainage until the time comes for detumescence. Finally, the man must be interested in having an erection and the various nerve pathways — both sensory and vasomotor — must be intact.

Testosterone is responsible for development of the genitalia, both *in utero* and at the time of puberty. Testosterone also determines libido: someone who is hypogonadal from childhood usually has little interest in sex, even though someone who is castrated as an adult may retain some drive and potency. Most men who present with impotence have normal libido, indicating that serum testosterone concentrations are likely to be normal. It follows that treatment with testosterone is illogical as well as ineffective — it heightens desire but does nothing for performance.

The autonomic nerve supply to the penis is not well understood. There are two efferent (erectogenic) pathways: the parasympathetic (S2, 3, 4; non-cholinergic) which is mainly responsible for reflex erections, and the sympathetic (T12/L1). The sympathetic pathway is non-adrenergic. The neurotransmitter is not known for either pathway. It may be vasoactive intestinal polypeptide (VIP), which is widely distributed in the nerve terminals of both the male and female genital tract.

There is also a sympathetic (adrenergic) anti-erectile pathway: sometimes the body finds an erection relatively inconvenient and needs to suppress it.

Impotence

Causes

The onset of erection failure is usually multifactorial. Psychological factors frequently contribute to its perpetuation, irrespective of the primary cause(s). A history may give clues as to psychosocial dysharmony, but other details (abrupt onset and intermittence) do not really help define a single cause. The major factors involved are listed in Table 11.1

Drugs

Spironolactone and digoxin are oestrogenic, while cimetidine and cyproterone acetate are antiandrogens. The mechanism for the impotence associated with β-blockade is not known. Thiazides may induce impotence by altering ionic distribution across the walls of the smooth muscles in arterioles and venules. Table 11.2 lists various drugs that may cause impotence.

Psychosocial causes

In general, doctors are too ready to diagnose psychogenic impotence: the majority of cases are mixed — both organic and psychogenic. On the other hand, premature ejaculation is usually psychosocial in its cause.

Ethanol

Excessive ethanol intake is associated with impotence, but the link is probably

Table 11.1. Factors involved in the pathogenesis of impotence

Atheroma
Neuropathy
   Sensory
   Efferent erectile pathways
   Vasomotor
Drugs: especially those used in hypertension (see Table 11.2)
Psychosocial factors
Ethanol abuse
Anatomical distortion of the penis

Table 11.2. Drugs associated with impotence

Thiazides
β-Blockers
Spironolactone
Digoxin
Cimetidine
Cyproterone acetate
Oestrogens

---

exaggerated. For most people ethanol is a disinhibitant and sexual stimulant. The links between ethanol and sexual failure are listed in Table 11.3. Note that the alcoholic male is unlikely to present with impotence *per se* (i.e. failure of erection but with intact libido), because libido will usually be lost as well.

Diabetes

Impotence is said to be more common also in diabetes. It probably is, affecting 30–50%, depending on age, but nobody knows the prevalence of impotence in non-diabetic males. The reason why diabetes may precipitate the problem may relate to the increased prevalence of neuropathy and vasculopathy in diabetes. It may also derive from some other fault (possibly a change in distribution of electrolytes across the cell walls of anteriolar smooth muscle). Such a mechanism would explain the occasional onset in young male diabetics before they have any other sign of neuropathy.

Assessment

1 Ensure that failure of erection is the real complaint.
2 Exclude obvious psychological and social problems.
3 Examine the man's genitalia (penis shape, testis size and consistency).
4 Measure testosterone (which should not be low), LH and prolactin (which should not be high). Even though endocrine causes are rare, they are easily excluded.
5 Refer for a trial of intracavernosal injection of a vasodilator, such as papaverine, without further investigation.

Table 11.3. Ethanol and sexual dysfunction

Ethanol-induced liver damage
    (increased serum oestrogen and increased sex hormone-binding globulin)
Testicular atrophy (low testosterone)
Hyperprolactinaemia (in acute intoxication)
Changes in fluid and electrolyte balance
Psychosocial (why does the man drink excessively anyway?)

Treatment

Explanation and reassurance

Many men and their partners are reasonably happy to accept the problem once it is all explained, and once they have had an opportunity to consider the various treatments. Reassurance must be informed, however, and it is not enough to find some bland phrase like 'What do you expect at your age?' or 'It happens to all men from time to time'. Alternative methods of deriving sexual satisfaction can be explained, if necessary.

Intracavernosal injections of papaverine

When self-administered, many otherwise impotent men achieve satisfactory erec-tions. People with neurogenic impotence (e.g. traumatic paraplegia) respond well, as do those with psychogenic causes, but those with bad vascular disease do not. There is risk of priapism, especially if too much is injected. Priapism is treated by either extraction of blood from the corpora with a 50 ml syringe, or by injection of the α-stimulant metaraminol.

Semi-rigid condom devices

Various devices are available and some couples find them acceptable, or at least better than nothing.

Penile implants

Semi-rigid rods can be implanted in the corpora cavernosa. More expensive models have tubes in the cavernosa which can have fluid pumped into them as required from an implanted sump, by squeezing a bulb in the scrotum: they are limp for most of the time, but a hydraulic erection can be achieved when desired.

Having considered the treatment options, it is easy to understand why many men are content to put with their problem.

Ejaculation

Ejaculation is usually preserved (indeed unwanted ejaculation can be a source of great distress in paraplegia). This means that successful intercourse is often possible if some means can be found to restore erections and achieve penetration. Retrograde ejaculation of semen into the bladder is an uncommon rare cause of subfertility in males, and may be caused by autonomic neuropathy.

MALE HYPOGONADISM

Hypogonadal males may have reduced spermatogenesis with or without reduced androgen secretion. Spermatogenesis is usually lost first.

Oligo- and azoospermia

Known causes of reduced spermatogenesis are shown in Table 11.4 but in most men with oligo- or azoospermia, the cause is obscure. They usually present with infertility. Histological examination gives no hint of a cause for the maturation arrest which is seen in the spermatocytes.

Table 11.4. Causes of oligo- or azoospermia

Congenital
Klinefelter's syndrome (47XXY)
Other chromosomal abnormalities
Maldescent of the testis

Acquired
Physical damage (irradiation, heat, surgery, infarction)
Infection (mumps in adulthood)
Cytotoxic drugs, ethanol
Liver disease
Treatment with oestrogens
Paraplegia
Haemochromatosis
Other possible unidentified environmental toxins

Endocrine
FSH deficiency
LH deficiency
Hyperprolactinaemia

Androgen deficiency

Causes

1 *Primary hypogonadism:* failure of the Leydig cells of the testis. Serum testosterone is low but serum LH is high because of reduced negative feedback inhibition.

2 *Secondary hypogonadism:* inadequate stimulation of the Leydig cells by LH, e.g. in people with a pituitary tumour or with idiopathic gonadotrophin-releasing hormone (GnRH) deficiency.

Clinical

The signs of androgen deficiency depend on the age at which they start. Someone who is hypogonadal from childhood will be eunuchoid (see Fig. 2.12), while someone who acquires hypogonadism in adulthood will be of normal stature. Both, however, will have other symptoms and signs of testosterone deficiency (Table 11.5).

Table 11.5. Symptoms of signs of testosterone deficiency

Reduced libido
Reduced growth of facial and body hair
Reduced temporal recession of capital hair
Reduced muscle bulk and skin thickness, fine wrinkled skin
Feminization: gynaecomastia and redistribution of body fat
Osteoporosis (loss of collagen in bone) with vertebral crush fractures

Treatment of hypogonadism

A man with hypogonadism will require treatment if he complains of reduced libido, reduced volume of semen, impotence or infertility. He should be treated in any case if he is young, because of the risk of prolonged androgen deficiency causing osteoporosis.

Treatment of cause

Causes which require treatment include structural disease of the hypothalamus and pituitary, hyperprolactinaemia and ethanol abuse.

Treatment of oligo- or azoospermia

Primary testicular defect

Treatment of infertility caused by primary failure of the seminiferous tubules rarely, if ever, works. Too little is known of the normal mechanisms and the reasons for their failure. The traditional recommendation concerning loose underpants and cold showers for azoospermic men represents a quaint approach with little scientific basis.

Although azoospermic or markedly oligospermic men should be told that they are almost certainly infertile, it is a mistake to be absolutely categorical. If the wife or partner does become pregnant at some stage, it is important to have allowed the possibility that the man is the father.

Realistically, the only effective remedy for a couple childless because of primary testicular disease is artificial insemination using donor semen (AID) or *in vitro* fertilization using donor semen.

Oligo- and azoospermia secondary to gonadotrophin deficiency

Treatment of secondary infertility (hypogonadism secondary to hypothalamic or pituitary disease) is possible. If the defect is hypothalamic (GnRH deficiency), it can be treated either with pulsatile infusions of GnRH, or with injections or exogenous gonadotrophins (see Fig. 2.14). If the hypogonadism is caused by pituitary disease with deficient LH and FSH, then treatment with GnRH is illogical and the treatment of choice is with injections of hCG (LH-like) and FSH. Treament is with two or three intramuscular injections for up to 6 months. If spermatogenesis is achieved, semen should be stored frozen for use by artificial insemination (AIH — husband's semen) next time.

Treatment of androgen deficiency

Steroids such as testosterone are well absorbed across the skin, and are stored in subcutaneous fat. Transdermal preparations are not yet widely available for replacement therapy in the male, but they may become standard therapy.

Oral androgens have to be taken two or three times daily, and are usually not as effective. Older preparations (methyl testosterone) had a tendency to cause cholestatic jaundice, but the risk of this seems low with modern preparations:

1 Mesterolone: 30–50 mg daily.
2 Restandol: testosterone undecanoate 40 mg, up to four each day.

However, higher serum testosterone concentrations are achieved with parenteral preparations. Monthly injections of testosterone esters (Sustanon or Primoteston) work well but are painful, and the effect on libido and sexual performance can reach unacceptable peaks after, and troughs before, each injection. They can be given in lower dosages more frequently.

For many men the best replacement therapy is with subcutaneous implants, 100–200 mg each 6–8 months.

Treatment of unsatisfactory sexual phenotype

Men may complain of physical attributes which they perceive as being undersized or abnormal. These include small penis, spindly physique, relative hairlessness. Such problems may be real or imagined (or a bit of both). Sadly, they are the result of natural variation in the population and endocrine investigation or treatment is rarely helpful. Most people know this and will accept reassurance, especially if it is cheered up with some line like 'little dogs often bark loudest'! Such cheerful reassurance should only be dispensed after the patient has been carefully questioned and examined.

TUMOURS OF THE TESTIS

Tumours of the testis are usually malignant: they represent approximately 1% of cancers in the male. The tumours derive from the different cellular elements of the testis — germ cells, Leydig cells, Sertoli cells and other tissues. Tumours of the germ cells are the most common, presumably because germ cells are constantly dividing and hence increasing the chance of mutations arising. This contrasts with the ovary (see p. 209): the germ cells of the ovary are not constantly dividing and germ cell tumours are relatively uncommon.

Germ-cell tumours

Seminoma

Seminomas occur in young men, aged 30–50 years. They are more frequent in maldescended or cryptorchid testes. Rarely, there may be a tumour on each side. Seminomas may be curable or may be highly malignant. There are a number of different histological types.

Teratoma

Teratomas of the testis are comprised of cells representing different embryonal cell layers: mesoderm, endoderm and ectoderm. They are highly malignant.

Chorioncarcinoma

Chorioncarcinomas and yolk-sac tumours occur. As in women, chorioncarcinomas secrete hCG, and this can cause thyrotoxicosis because hCG has weak thyroid-stimulating hormone (TSH)-like activity.

Sex-cord tumours (tumours of gonadal stroma)

Leydig-cell tumour

These are usually benign and curable by excision. They secrete both androgens and oestrogens: affected men present with symptoms and signs of feminization.

Sertoli-cell tumour

These are very rare. They may secrete either androgens or oestrogens.

GYNAECOMASTIA

The breast is made up of glandular tissue and fat. Glandular tissue increases in size and activity when exposed to oestrogens (but requires other hormones, including growth hormone and thyroxine, as well). Androgens antagonize the action of oestrogens on the breast. The fatty tissue is also under the control of oestrogens to some extent.

Causes

Puberty gynaecomastia

About 50% of boys develop enlargement of the breast tissue as they go through puberty. It may be embarrassing or painful, or they may fleetingly fear they have breast cancer. It usually goes away. If it persists and is gross, the only recognized treatment is with plastic surgery (reduction mammoplasty), but this can leave an unsightly scar. Treatment with oral antioestrogens such as danazol or tamoxifen has been advocated but there is no published evidence of their effectiveness.

Gynaecomastia in adults

Most men with enlarged breasts are simply fat. However, some have true breast enlargement — both glandular and fatty — because of endocrine factors. These factors are:

1 Relative excess of oestrogen.
   (a) Oestrogen treatment (e.g. carcinoma of the prostate, transsexuals).
   (b) Increased oestrone production in chronic hepatic disease.
   (c) Increased oestrogen production by testes which are failing.
   (d) Administration of drugs with oestrogenic actions: spironolactone, digoxin.
   (e) Increased synthesis of oestrogens by aromatization of androgens in peripheral tissue, especially in fatter people. This may also be the mechanism for the gynaecomastia which can complicate illicit androgen therapy in body-builders.
   (f) Oestrogen-secreting tumour of the testis or adrenal.
   (g) Thyrotoxicosis (probably because of the increase in sex hormone binding globulin which occurs).
2 Relative deficiency of androgens: primary hypogonadism, for example that complicates Klinefelter's syndrome, or mumps orchitis.
3 Target organ insensitivity to androgens:
   (a) Administration of drugs with antiandrogenic actions: cyproterone acetate, cimetidine.

(b) Syndromes of androgen insensitivity.

(c) It is possible that many cases of idiopathic gynaecomastia are the result of relative tissue insensitivity to androgens, but this is speculative.

4 Unknown mechanism.

Gynaecomastia can occur in lung cancers, but the reason is not known.

Investigation

Puberty gynaecomastia is the commonest cause, and the second most common is probably body-building, with or without steroid abuse. In many cases there is no obvious cause. The principles of examination and investigation are:

1 Exclude the very rare possibility of carcinoma.

2 Exclude obvious causes of gynaecomastia, such as drugs, hypogonadism or liver disease.

3 Measure serum oestradiol to exclude occult (and very rare) oestrogen-secreting tumours.

Prolactin excess does *not* cause gynaecomastia. It causes milk secretion in the oestrogen-primed breast.

Chapter 12
Female Sexual Function —
Gynaecological Endocrinology

THE OVARY

The ovary has two functions: the production of ova, and the production of sex steroids (androgens and oestrogens).

Development

Unlike the testis, the ovary remains relatively undifferentiated until the 5th month of gestation, when primitive granulosa cells become arranged around the dividing oocytes to form primordial follicles. At the same time, other cells have developed the enzymes necessary for steroidogenesis.

The Mullerain duct persists to form the Fallopian tubes and uterus. The Wolffian system does not develop (see Fig. 10.2).

Anatomy

The ovaries are ovoid, each about 3.5 cm in length and weighing 4–8 g. Nerves, vessels and lymphatics enter at the hilum (Fig. 12.1). The right ovarian vein drains directly into the inferior vena cava, while the left ovarian vein drains into the left renal vein. The ovaries lie at the back of the broad ligaments, and are the only intra-abdominal structures which are not covered by peritoneum.

The ripening ovum lies within a follicle lined by several layers of granulosa cells. The stromal cells surrounding the follicle form a false capsule (the theca interna). After ovulation the follicle forms the corpus luteum, before becoming atretic. The functional organization within the ovarian stroma is complex — undoubtedly much more so than is currently understood.

Theca cells

The cells of the theca interna synthesize androgens, principally androstenedione and testosterone. Serum testosterone concentrations in women are between 0.8 and 2.7 nmol litre^{-1} (10–30% of male values). However, most testosterone is probably used locally within the ovary, because it is the precursor for synthesis of oestradiol (E_2), the main female sex hormone.

Granulosa cells

The granulosa cells are those which line the ripening ovarian follicle. They utilize testosterone from the theca interna, and synthesize E_2. Circulating E_2 (between 200 and 1000 pmol litre^{-1}, 0.2–1.0 nmol litre^{-1}) in the follicular phase of the menstrual cycle prepares vaginal and cervical mucus for sperm penetration, and the endometrium for implantation of a fertilized ovum.

The granulosa cells also synthesize peptide hormones, including inhibin and insulin-like growth factors (IGFs). Inhibin is a two-chain polypeptide which

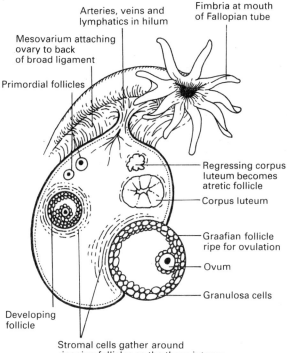

Fig. 12.1. Structure of the ovary.

feeds back on the pituitary to reduce follicle-stimulating hormone (FSH) (but not luteinizing hormone (LH)) secretion. FSH stimulates the formation of IGF_1 by the granulosa cells and this augments the action of FSH on E_2 synthesis (Fig. 12.2).

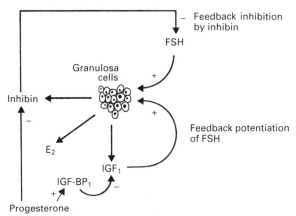

Fig. 12.2. Some of the more complex hormonal interactions in the granulosa cell of the Graafian follicle. After ovulation, progesterone is secreted by the corpus luteum. It stimulates production of IGF binding protein ($IGF-BP_1$) which inactivates IGF_1.

Corpus luteum

The ripe ovarian follicle releases its ovum when it is up to 2 cm in diameter. The residual cells of the follicle reform into the corpus luteum. The function of the corpus luteum is to support the ovum in the early days after fertilization and implantation into the endometrium, before the placenta is established. To do this, the biochemical function of the granulosa cells alters critically. Instead of producing E_2, the main steroid secreted is progesterone (see Fig. 1.11). Progesterone also acts on the breast to stimulate glandular development, and is responsible for the breast engorgement felt by ovulating women in the later stages of the menstrual cycle.

Progesterone inactivates IGF_1 by stimulating synthesis of its binding protein $IGF\text{-}BP_1$ within the ovary. It also inhibits the secretion of inhibin, allowing FSH to rise at the beginning of the next menstrual cycle — assuming that conception does not occur (see Fig. 12.2).

The corpus luteum also secretes the peptide hormone relaxin. The function of relaxin in early pregnancy is not known, but it is so-called because of its ability to allow the relaxation and stretching of the symphysis pubis which occurs during vaginal delivery. Relaxin is structurally related to insulin and IGFs.

The menstrual cycle

Follicle-stimulating hormone is secreted as circulating concentrations of progesterone and inhibin fall in the luteal phase of the preceding cycle. It stimulates the maturation of (usually) a single dominant ovarian follicle, in one or other ovary. The ripening follicle secretes inhibin, which suppresses FSH by negative feedback. The ripening follicle also secretes E_2, and this provokes a surge of release of LH at mid-cycle (Fig. 12.3). This positive feedback effect of oestrogen on LH secretion occurs only in women; in men, LH secretion is suppressed by oestrogens. The mid-cycle LH burst stimulates ovulation: the ovum floats into the

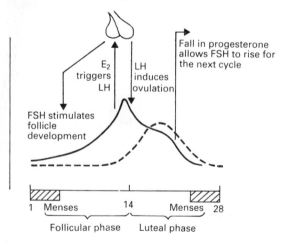

Fig. 12.3. Hormonal changes during the menstrual cycle. E_2, ——; progesterone, – – –

Fallopian tube, while the remaining granulosa cells form the corpus luteum. The corpus luteum secretes progesterone to support any early pregnancy. However, if fertilization and implantation do not occur, the corpus luteum starts to involute and progesterone secretion falls.

Oestradiol stimulates proliferation of the endometrium; IGF_1 is also involved. The production of progesterone in the luteal phase stimulates production of $IGF\text{-}BP_1$ in the endometrium, and this halts the proliferation induced by IGF_1. The endometrium is shed as progesterone concentrations fall. There are complex endocrine interactions between the ovary and uterus, but they are only dimly understood.

The menopause

The ovaries stop producing ova and sex steroids after 30–40 years. The reason for this is not known: the supply of ova is not exhausted, but the ovaries become resistant to stimulation by gonadotrophins. Basal FSH concentrations in serum rise first, followed by LH. Despite high basal concentrations, both are still secreted in bursts. Bursts of LH and FSH secretion are linked to the 'hot flushes' of the menopausal years.

Hot flushes

Luteinizing hormone and FSH do not cause the flushes because their rise follows the start of the flush, rather than the other way round. Presumably both are triggered by an unidentified alteration in hypothalamic neurotransmitter release. The neurotransmitter may be an opioid peptide, dopamine, a catecholamine, or all three. Hot flushes can be attenuated by oral oestrogens, by sympathetic antagonists such as clonidine, and — under experimental conditions — by injection of opioid receptor blockers such as naloxone. Hot flushes wane with time, but LH and FSH levels remain high.

Hypogonadism following the menopause

As the ovaries fail, ovulation ceases and sex steroid production declines. The fall in oestrogens leads to regression of the secondary sexual characteristics: loss of breast and other body fat, sometimes a change from female to male-pattern hair growth, and loss of the protective effect of oestrogens on atherogenesis. Falling oestrogenic stimulation of vaginal secretion may cause dryness and discomfort with intercourse (dyspareunia). This in itself may cause reduced libido, but sex drive may also fall with a decline in androgen secretion. Reduced secretion of oestrogens and androgens leads also to loss of the collagen matrix of bone and osteoporosis. This bone loss is progressive.

Post-menopausal osteoporosis is less likely in women who have had pregnancies, are plumper and who have a later menopause. It is more likely in those who are nulliparous, thin and who go through the menopause at a relatively young age. It is common in Caucasians, but very rare in Afro-Caribbeans. The tendency to bone loss may be exacerbated by various other factors, including thyroid disease, lack of physical exercise and ethanol abuse.

Premature ovarian failure

Some women undergo an early menopause. This can occur in the teenage years, and can even be a cause of primary amenorrhoea. Sometimes (uncommonly) antiovarian antibodies can be demonstrated, but usually there is no obvious reason. It cannot be treated.

Resistant ovary syndrome

Rarely, a woman can present with the clinical and biochemical features of premature menopause, but have the resistant ovary syndrome. The ovaries become resistant to the action of FSH and/or LH because of some undefined receptor abnormality. It can be transient, or it can persist.

Hormone replacement therapy

Hormone replacement therapy (HRT) is used increasingly widely to replace the oestrogen which is lost as the woman goes through the menopause. Its advantages are:

1 Reduced likelihood of osteoporosis.
2 Reduced likelihood of cardiovascular disease.
3 Preservation of secondary sexual characteristics.
4 Suppression of menopausal symptoms, including 'hot flushes'.

HRT also seems to attenuate some of the psychological sequelae that accompany the menopause.

It seems reasonable to offer HRT to all women who are likely to benefit from it: those with symptoms, those whose menopause is early, and those whose serum E_2 concentration is shown to be low. It is difficult to be dogmatic about side-effects: the doses of oestrogen are generally lower, and hence the contraindications are not necessarily the same as for the combined oral contraceptive. Thus obesity, cigarette smoking and migraine remain only relative contraindications.

Hypertension, diabetes and vascular disease are not necessarily contraindications: low-dose oestrogens are likely to have a protective effect, if anything. The only definite contraindications are hormone-dependent carcinoma, endometriosis, hepatic disease, previous thromboembolism and unacceptable symptomatic side-effects.

Conventional hormone replacement therapy has to be given cyclically in women who still have a uterus, because unopposed oestrogen therapy can cause endometrial hyperplasia and this can be premalignant. Newer preparations, e.g. tibolone, are available for continuous use — and do not cause withdrawal bleeds. There are a number of packeted cyclical preparations available, although prescription charges can be illogically expensive for some of them because the charge is doubled if the preparation contains two separate compounds. Oestrogens can also be administered trans-dermally (steroids are well absorbed across the skin), vaginally, or by subcutaneous implant. Vaginal and vulval creams are available for dryness and dyspareunia.

Therapy is most beneficial if it is started before oestrogen levels fall. There is no agreement on how long HRT should be continued.

DISEASES OF THE OVARY AND ABNORMALITIES OF OVARIAN FUNCTION

Ovarian agenesis

Agenesis occurs either in isolation or as a manifestation of chromosomal disorders, such as Turner's syndrome.

Treatment

The woman requires HRT to achieve normal secondary sexual development, and to avoid the consequences of oestrogen deficiency.

Ovarian neoplasia

Most ovarian tumours are derived from epithelial cells (80% +), or germ cells (5% +). They do not secrete hormones and are more likely to present to a gynaecologist rather than an endocrinologist. However, those derived from stromal/sex-cord cells (10%), such as granulosa and hilus-cell tumours, can present as a result of hormone secretion. They may present with hirsutism and high testosterone levels. Testosterone concentrations are usually very high (> 5 nmol litre^{-1}).

Polycystic ovary syndrome

The small ovarian cysts which are often found in this condition are the result of the problem, not the cause. Not all women with the polycystic ovary syndrome (PCO) have cysts. The name of the condition is a poor one, but the pathogenesis is so complex that it has not been possible to find a better one.

Pathogenesis

Polycystic ovary syndrome is a complex hormonal disorder: the cyclical servo-mechanism which controls ovarian function is upset. There is no definite single cause — it could be any or all of the following (Fig. 12.4):

1 Abnormal patterns of LH release.
2 Abnormal secretion of androgens by adrenal or ovary or both.
3 Excessive ovarian inhibin secretion, caused by increased androgens and resulting in suppressed FSH secretion and defective follicle development.
4 Defective hepatic synthesis of sex hormone-binding globulin (SHBG), causing abnormal androgen transport in serum.
5 Increased androgens being aromatized to oestrogens (especially in the adipocytes, and especially in fatter people), with the oestrogens increasing pituitary secretion of LH and prolactin.
6 Insulin resistance and abnormal IGF synthesis, causing reduced SHBG synthesis and increased androgen synthesis by the ovary.
7 Obesity — which might be a cause, e.g. by causing insulin resistance, or an exacerbating factor, or even a consequence of the condition. Low-density lipoproteins stimulate androgen synthesis.

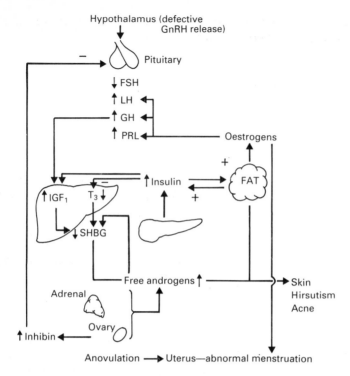

Fig. 12.4. Some of the factors involved in the polycystic ovary syndrome complex. PRL, prolactin; SHBG, sex hormone-binding globulin.

Clinical

This complex and ill-understood condition may present in a number of different ways:
1 Hirsutism and acne.
2 Irregular menstruation (usually infrequent, rather than excessive).
3 Infertility (from anovulation).
4 Galactorrhoea (from hyperprolactinaemia).
5 Obesity.

Not surprisingly, there is associated lack of self-esteem and depression. Depression and feelings of rejection are exacerbated by doctors who find the condition difficult to understand and difficult to treat.

Diagnosis

The diagnosis is mainly clinical. However, suggestive biochemical confirmation is provided by demonstrating:
1 High normal or slightly high serum total testosterone.
2 Reduced serum SHBG (< 40 nmol litre^{-1}).
3 Highish LH and lowish FSH.
4 Highish serum prolactin (only in some).

Ultrasound of the ovaries may reveal multiple (> 5), small (< 1 cm) cysts but these are no more invariable than any other features of this protean problem. Multiple small cysts also occur in normal women.

Treatment

Treatment depends on the dominant symptom.

Hirsutism

The treatment of hirsutism is discussed in detail below.

Infertility

It is usually possible to induce ovulation with clomiphene. Alternatively, treatment with low doses of corticosteroids (e.g. 5.0 mg prednisolone daily) may be effective. The corticosteroids suppress adrenal androgen synthesis.

Galactorrhoea

Hyperprolactinaemia can be corrected by treatment with a dopamine receptor agonist such as bromocriptine.

Obesity

There is no alternative to calorie restriction, but diets in obese people with PCO can be depressingly ineffective — possibly linked to hyperinsulinism and abnormal thermogenesis (see p. 165). When diets prove ineffective, both patient and doctor become frustrated. The patient blames the doctor for lack of effective treatment, and the doctor blames the patient for being 'non-compliant' (i.e. weak-willed and greedy).

Amenorrhoea

Chronic unopposed action of oestrogens causes endometrial proliferation without regular shedding. This causes oligomenorrhoea and amenorrhoea. There is also a threefold risk of developing endometrial malignancy. Monthly treatment with a progestogen (e.g. medroxyprogesterone acetate 5 mg daily for 5 days) induces regular withdrawal bleeding and this reduces the risk of carcinoma.

Hirsutism

Hirsutism is the complaint by a woman of excessive facial and body hair. It may be accompanied by loss of capital hair, and/or by acne. There may be associated virilism — increased muscle bulk and more masculine physique, clitoral enlargement, deepening voice.

Hirsutism results from an interaction between serum androgens, which may or may not be elevated, and hair follicles, which are more sensitive to circulating androgens. Elevated androgens actually induce increased sensitivity in target organs by increasing the activity of the enzyme which converts testosterone to DHT — 5α-reductase.

Causes

1   Androgen-secreting tumours of the ovary or adrenal (rare: 1% of cases).

2 Cushing's syndrome (equally rare).
3 Congenital adrenal hyperplasia (CAH).
4 Androgen therapy — in athletes, and those being treated with androgens or anabolic steroids.
5 Some progestogen preparations, e.g. in the combined oral contraceptive.
6 Other drugs, e.g. phenytoin, cyclosporin, diazoxide, minoxidil.
7 PCO.
8 Unexplained — presumably caused by abnormal skin sensitivity to normal concentrations of circulating androgens.

Racial factors

Women of Mediterranean extraction and those who are racially Indian may have more body hair than north Europeans. However, such women are just as likely to suffer from PCO or some other endocrine disorder, and it is a mistake to dismiss their complaint of hirsutism as being 'racial'. An Indian woman is more likely than a Caucasian doctor to know whether or not her hair growth is excessive.

Investigation

1 Testosterone — if it is greater than 5 nmol litre^{-1}, there is a 20% chance of the woman having an androgen-secreting tumour.
2 Prolactin — women with high levels may be treated with bromocriptine.
3 17-OHP — to exclude CAH.
4 SHBG.

Treatment

An essential aspect of management is explanation and reassurance. This is all that some women want. Other approaches are:
1 *Cosmetic:*
   (a) Depilatory creams (not very effective and cause skin rashes).
   (b) Plucking (painful but effective).
   (c) Waxing (good for abdomen and thighs).
   (d) Electrolysis (used mainly on face; expensive, better in milder cases).
   (e) Bleaching (makes dark hairs less obvious).
   (f) Shaving. (Causes a blow to self-esteem, but does *not* make hair growth worse, as is often claimed. It does, however, leave a sharp stubble.)
2 *Dietary:* if a woman can lose weight, it may reduce insulin resistance and improve the problem. It will certainly increase self-esteem.
3 *Hormonal:* hormonal manipulation should be saved for those who are likely to respond, i.e. those who have an identifiable abnormality such as high testosterone or low SHBG. Possible complications should be carefully explained. Obesity, hypertension, migraine, thromboembolism and symptomatic side-effects are contraindications. The options are:
   (a) Oestrogens: these have to be given cyclically, in combination with a progestogen, unless the woman has had a hysterectomy. They act directly on the skin as antiandrogens. They also stimulate SHBG synthesis in the liver.

When serum SHBG is higher, the concentration of circulating androgen which is free, is lower.

(b) Spironolactone: spironolactone is an oestrogen (as well as an aldosterone antagonist), and is effective in hirsutism. Unfortunately its use is not recommended by the Committee on the Safety of Medicines.

(c) Antiandrogens: cyproterone acetate is a very potent antiandrogen (decreasing androgen synthesis and antagonizing their actions on the skin). It helps hair growth in approximately 50% of cases. Although cyproterone acetate has been used for 15 years, knowledge of its long-term side-effects is limited.

Premenstrual syndrome

Some women feel unwell in the days leading up to menstruation, sometimes severely so. Symptoms are various: bloatedness, breast tenderness, abdominal pain, depression, irritability, etc. There is no known link between the premenstrual syndrome and any known abnormality of hormone secretion, and hormonal therapy is rarely successful. The administration of a combined contraceptive preparation often makes the symptoms worse. It is likely that some women rationalize non-specific malaise and symptoms by linking them to menstruation, and have, therefore, no specific gynaecological problem. However, it is also likely that others do have some abnormality — hormonal or otherwise — which is simply not understood. There is no specific treatment. Encouragement and understanding are all that orthodox medicine can offer. Many women derive benefit from homoeopathy, hypnotherapy and herbal medicines.

Oligomenorrhoea, secondary amenorrhoea and anovulation

Oligomenorrhoea (periods each 35 days to 6 months) and secondary amenorrhoea (periods more than 6 months apart) are the result of defective cyclical function of the ovary. Primary amenorrhoea may also be the result of major developmental abnormalities of the ovary and uterus.

Causes

As normal cyclical function involves so many different factors, there are many possible ways in which it can go wrong. Diagnosis is by a process of elimination:

1 Severe systemic disease or trauma, leading to defective release of hypothalamic GnRH.

2 Gross weight loss — most commonly from anorexia nervosa in the UK, and from starvation worldwide. Restoration of periods can be delayed for up to 2 years after ideal body weight is regained.

3 Hypothalamic or pituitary disease with LH and FSH deficiency.

4 Hyperprolactinaemia — is associated with defective LH and FSH secretion.

5 Hyperthyroidism.

6 PCO and hyperandrogenism.

7 Post-partum — the length of the amenorrhoea is longer if the woman is breastfeeding.

8 Post-pill — menstrual irregularity should persist for no more than 6 months.

   9 Menopause.
   10 Unexplained.

Investigation of oligo- or amenorrhoea

After taking a history and examination, the following should help define treatable causes:

1 Weight/body mass index.
2 Full blood count and erythrocyte sedimentation rate.
3 Thyroid function tests.
4 Prolactin.
5 LH and FSH.
6 Testosterone, SHBG.

Diagnosis of anovulation in women with regular periods

Some women may have regular periods without ovulating regularly. This can be demonstrated by:

1 Loss of normal biphasic change in basal body temperature (tedious and imprecise).
2 Serum progesterone concentration < 40 nmol litre^{-1} at days 20–22 of a 28-day cycle.
3 Absence of full follicle development on sequential scanning of the ovaries by ultrasound.

Short luteal phase

Some women with short menstrual cycles have a luteal phase which is less than 14 days. This may be insufficient to allow the successful implantation of a fertilized embryo. The endocrine basis of this condition is not clear.

Menorrhagia

Menorrhagia is not usually the result of a hormonal problem. The only condition which should be excluded is hypothyroidism.

INFERTILITY

A couple who have been trying to achieve a pregnancy for 12 months or more may be said to be subfertile. Of those referred to an infertility clinic at this stage, 80% will achieve a pregnancy after a further 12 months. Infertility may be primary (no preceding pregnancy) or secondary. Infertility is generally taken to mean failure of conception or implantation, rather than recurrent abortion.

Causes

Coital

Five per cent of couples complaining of infertility have some problems of coitus. Ignorance about sexual intercouse is relatively uncommon, but still occurs. Infrequency of sexual intercourse can be significant, and a request for help with infertility is sometimes a prelude to the collapse of a relationship.

Semen and mucus

A sperm count of < 20 million ml^{-1} is thought to be subnormal and a contributory factor to infertility, but many men father children with counts less than this. Total sperm count is also variable, being rather lower for 1 or 2 days following ejaculation. The lower the total count, and the higher the percentage of abnormal forms with impaired motility *in vitro*, the greater the chance that the man is responsible. The ability of the spermatozoa to penetrate mucus *in vitro* can be documented semi-quantitatively (sperm invasion test), as can the persistence of live spermatozoa in the cervical mucus taken from the woman after sexual intercourse (post-coital test).

Female genital tract

Apart from congenital anomalies, the passage may be blocked by the effects of previous pelvic inflammatory disease, or by endometriosis.

Anovulation

Fertilization will not occur without ovulation. This means more than just the release of an ovum: the ovum has to be released in a receptive state. Similarly, the genital tract has to be receptive to implantation of the implanted embryo. Gonadal steroids (oestrogens and progesterone) are important, but so too are a host of peptide growth factors and prostaglandins.

Sometimes ovulation is followed by a relatively short luteal phase (< 12 days). The mechanism is not known, but it is thought that failure of the corpus luteum may leave the newly implanted embryo without protection.

Management

Failure to conceive is a source of great potential distress, and should be managed by experts with precision and efficiency. It is usually managed badly. It is managed best with continuity (i.e. by the same doctor), and by staff who are fully trained. All too often, couples who suffer with infertility return repeatedly to a gynaecological clinic at 3-monthly intervals to see a junior doctor who is not a specialist in infertility management and whom they have never met before. Given the inherent invasion of privacy of the process, this leads to major distress, which is usually underestimated by professionals.

Once such supervision has been ensured, the next stage is the definition of the strategy of management. The strategy will vary from couple to couple. It should be agreed with them, and written down.

1 History and examination of both partners, including semen analysis.

2 Explanation and reassurance, including agreement on strategy.

3 Definition of ovulation.

4 Sperm invasion test.

5 Definition of patency of female genital tract (laparoscopy or hysterosalpingogram).

6 Treatment: induction of ovulation, *in vitro* fertilization (IVF), intraFallopian transfer of gamete (GIFT), artificial insemination using husband or donor semen (AIH, AID).

7 Agreeing when to stop trying.

8 Advice on adoption.

Induction of ovulation

Clomiphene

If a woman is not ovulating regularly, she can be treated with clomiphene. This is an oestrogen-antagonist which causes the hypothalamus to release FSH and LH. Fifty to 150 mg are given orally for 5 days at the beginning of each cycle if the woman is menstruating, or monthly if she is not. Clomiphene is usually given on days 5–10, and the response of the ovarian follicles is documented by ultrasound. If there is a single dominant follicle, an additional injection of hCG (which is like LH) is sometimes given on day 12, 13 or 14. In PCO it is sometimes possible to restore menstruation and ovulation with low-dose corticosteroids (e.g. 5.0 mg prednisolone).

GnRH

Ovulation can also be induced in women with defective LH and FSH release by pulsatile subcutaneous administration of GnRH during the follicular phase of the cycle. The woman has an indwelling cannula, and carries a syringe driver in a small holster. If the GnRH is not given in pulses about 90 min apart, the LH and FSH rise too high for too long and this induces ovarian resistance.

Gonadotrophins

Women with disease of the pituitary (e.g. a previous tumour) and gonadotrophin deficiency may need injections of gonadotrophins if they are gonadotrophin-deficient. Daily injections of 75–225 U human menopausal gonadotrophin (HMG, extracted from the urine of post-menopausal women) in the follicular phase acts like FSH, and hCG may be given (500–1500 U i.m.) in mid-cycle if the development of a single dominant follicle is demonstrated on ultrasound (see Fig. 2.14). Human chorionic gonadotrophin should not be given if there are multiple follicles because of the risk of inducing multiple ovulation and multiple pregnancy.

Gonadotrophins in combination with GnRH analogues

An alternative strategy is sometimes tried when the ovary is resistant to stimulation by exogenous gonadotrophins. Thus, gonadotrophins may be given after the secretion of endogenous LH and FSH has been suppressed by intranasal administration of a GnRH analogue, such as buserelin. Such a stategy is used also for programming timed ovulation prior to IVF and GIFT.

ENDOCRINOLOGY OF PREGNANCY

Corpus luteum

If the ovum is fertilized, the corpus luteum persists — possibly being maintained by hCG from the embryo. The corpus luteum is the source of progesterone in the early weeks of pregnancy, but is not clear how this ensures survival of the fetus. The corpus luteum starts to shrink from the 10th week, but persists until term.

Fertilized ovum and decidua

The fertilized ovum expresses hormone receptors (for insulin and IGFs, as well as others) as early as the 4- and 8-cell stages. It also secretes growth factors, which facilitate implantation.

Placental hormones

The placenta synthesizes a host of peptide hormones. The best recognized are hCG and human placental lactogen. Human chorionic gonadotrophin ensures persistence of the corpus luteum. Peak hCG production occurs at about 10 weeks, and it declines to low levels after the 16th week. It is structurally related to TSH, and there is evidence that it assumes control of the thyroid gland in the first trimester (see below).

Human placental lactogen is related to GH, and is a growth factor. Its precise role in facilitating fetal growth and development is not clear. It is secreted in massive quantities (approximately 1 g day^{-1}) in the third trimester.

Fetoplacental hormones

Oestrogens and progesterone levels are both high in pregnancy. In the early weeks they derive from the ovary, but they are later synthesized by the placenta, using dehydroepiandrosterone sulphate (DHEAS) from the fetal adrenal as a precursor. The first stage of conversion is desulphation to DHEA (dehydroepiandrosterone) and this is dependent on the presence of placental sulphatase. Placental sulphatase deficiency is an uncommon X-linked recessive disorder (nearly always affecting only male pregnancies) in which the desulphation of DHEAS is limited, and pregnancy oestrogens are very low. Affected children are usually delivered by Caesarean section, but the pregnancy is otherwise uneventful.

Prolactin

Maternal serum prolactin concentrations rise to high levels throughout pregnancy (up to $20\,000 \text{ mU litre}^{-1}$). This rise is due to the stimulation of pituitary lactotrophs by high circulating oestrogen concentrations. Prolactin probably acts as a growth factor, but its main recognized action is the facilitation of lactation. It is necessary for the start of lactation, but not for its maintenance.

Fetal prolactin secretion is also high, and prolactin is secreted by the cells of the amnion into amniotic fluid.

The thyroid in pregnancy

The thyroid of the mother undergoes major changes in pregnancy, partly as a result of hCG production, and partly as a result of the changes in autoimmune processes that occur. Assessment of thyroid function in pregnancy can, however, be extremely difficult. This is partly because oestrogens stimulate thyroid-binding globulin synthesis, causing a high serum thyroxine concentration, and partly because TSH may be undetectable in up to 50% of normal pregnancies in the first trimester (see below). The only reliable way to diagnose thyrotoxicosis in early pregnancy is with an assay of free thyroxine, and even that is method-dependent.

Effects of hCG

Human chorionic gonadotrophin stimulates the thyroid and the secretion of pituitary TSH is lessened in the first trimester — when hCG concentrations are highest. There is a suggestion that severe vomiting in pregnancy (hyperemesis gravidarum) may sometimes be caused by hCG-induced thyrotoxicosis.

Alterations in the immune system

The immune system of women is relatively suppressed during pregnancy: auto-immune diseases tend to go into remission. This includes autoimmune diseases of the thyroid, such as Graves' disease. However, this remission is often followed by rebound reactivation.

In recent years it has been recognized that a specific autoimmune disorder of the thyroid may complicate pregnancy: painless post-partum thyroiditis. Thus it has been demonstrated that approximately 15% of women have a rise in antithy-roid microsomal antibodies in the months after delivery, and that this rise in antibodies is followed by transient hyperthyroidism, or hypothyroidism, or both. The condition is usually self-limiting. It is not known whether the 15% of women who have thyroid dysfunction in the 12 months after delivery are the same 15% who suffer with post-partum depression, but it seems possible.

Chapter 13
Calcium Metabolism and Disorders of Bone

CALCIUM METABOLISM

Calcium, magnesium and phosphate are essential for life. Calcium mediates the majority of intracellular messages (see Second messengers, pp. 22–4), and a normal blood calcium concentration is essential for normal depolarization of nerve and muscle cell membranes, as well as for blood clotting. Magnesium shares some of the actions of calcium, but the relationships between the two are not well understood. Phosphate is an essential component of cell walls, and the key ion in intracellular energy generation. Phosphate ions in blood buffer calcium and magnesium, as well as other cations.

Calcium homoeostasis

As calcium and phosphate are major constituents of bone and of all cells, it follows that there is a vast body pool of them. Moreover, they are abundant in food and there is usually little tendency for the body to be short of them. They are ingested in excess, and the surplus is excreted from the bowel and in the urine. The role of the body's homoeostatic mechanisms are therefore aimed primarily at buffering the peaks that occur after meals and smoothing the troughs between them.

There are three main homoeostatic mechanisms (Fig. 13.1):

1 Control of absorption of calcium from the bowel, mainly by 1,25-OHCC (1,25-dihydroxycholecalciferol, vitamin D).

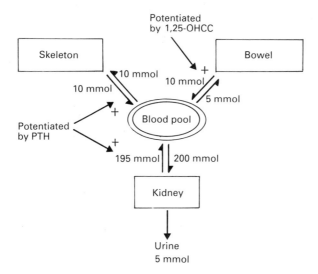

Fig. 13.1. Calcium homeostasis. PTH, parathyroid hormone.

Table 13.1. Correction of total serum albumin

For every gram the albumin is below 40 g litre^{-1}, add 0.02 mmol litre^{-1} to the measured calcium. For every gram the albumin is above 40 g litre^{-1}, subtract 0.02.

Example:

Measured calcium	1.90 mmol litre^{-1}
Albumin	22 g litre^{-1}
Corrected calcium	1.90 + 18 (i.e. 40 – 22) × 0.02 = 2.26 mmol litre^{-1} (normal)

Corrected total serum calcium should lie between 2.20 and 2.60 mmol litre^{-1}

2   Control of renal reabsorption of calcium which has been filtered into the renal tubule, mainly by parathyroid hormone (PTH).
3   Increased release of calcium from bone to maintain circulating calcium concentrations, mainly by PTH.
Under normal circumstances the dietary intake of calcium (approximately 25 mmol day^{-1}) is sufficient to balance the loss in urine (5 mmol) and faeces (20 mmol). If small adjustments are required they are made by changing calcium reabsorption in the renal tubule. Although the pool of calcium in bones is enormous (1 kg calcium in the bones of a 70 kg man), it does not contribute much to normal day-to-day control of calcium homoeostasis. It only becomes significant when there is
1   dietary deficiency of calcium;
2   dietary deficiency of vitamin D;
3   dysfunction of either the parathyroids or the kidneys.
Serum calcium is bound to a number of serum proteins, but mainly to albumin. It is the unbound, ionized fraction (55% total) which is active. Most laboratories measure total, rather than ionized, calcium but the results are affected by changes in serum albumin concentration. For these reasons it is usual to apply a correction factor (calcium corrected to normal albumin) to total calcium. It assumes a normal albumin concentration of 40 g litre^{-1} (Table 13.1).

Vitamin D

The structure and metabolism of vitamin D is described on pp. 13–15. Ten per cent is derived from dietary ergocalciferol (vitamin D_2) and 90% from cholecalciferol (vitamin D_3) produced from 7-dehydrocholesterol in skin under the influence of sunlight. Cholecalciferol is activated by being 25-hydroxylated in the liver, and 1α-hydroxylated in the kidneys to produce dihydroxycholecalciferol (1,25-OHCC). 1,25-OHCC is produced when serum calcium concentrations show a tendency to fall. When calcium concentrations are high, 1,25-OHCC synthesis is reduced and the inactive isomer 24,25-OHCC is synthesized in the kidneys instead (see Fig. 1.10).
The main action of 1,25-OHCC is to increase the intestinal absorption of calcium. It acts by entering the nuclei of intestinal epithelial cells and stimulating the production of mRNA directly.

The parathyroid glands

There are normally four parathyroid glands in humans. They are usually found on the posterior surface of the upper and lower poles of each lobe of the thyroid, but their position is very variable. Total weight is approximately 120 g.

There are two sorts of cell in the parathyroid: the chief cell, which secretes PTH, and the oxyphil cell. The function of the oxyphil cell is not known; it first appears at the time of puberty and numbers slowly increase throughout life.

PTH

Parathyroid hormone (84 amino acids) is derived from enzymic cleavage of prepro-PTH (115 amino acids) and pro-PTH (90 amino acids). Its half-life in serum is approximately 20 minutes, but a number of inactive degradation products may be detected by radioimmunoassay.

Parathyroid hormone is secreted in response to a fall in ionized calcium, and acts mainly on bone and on the kidney tubule. It interacts with specific cell-surface receptors, and stimulates cyclic adenosine monophosphate (cAMP) production. In the kidney it stimulates calcium and H^+ ion reabsorption, and the excretion of phosphate and bicarbonate. It has a biphasic action on bone, inducing the short-term release of calcium and phosphate, and stimulating osteoclast differentiation.

C-cells (parafollicular cells) of the thyroid

Although these cells are scattered throughout the thyroid, they have no known functional relationship with thyroid hormones. They secrete calcitonin. In some species, but not in humans, calcitonin lowers serum calcium concentration by inhibiting osteoclasts — and acts as a PTH antagonist. In humans, calcitonin has no known physiological action. Serum calcium is normal in medullary carcinoma of the thyroid (carcinoma of the C-cells), even though serum calcitonin production may be very high. None the less, calcitonin is sometimes used therapeutically in the treatment of hypercalcaemia and of Paget's disease.

Two other hormones are very closely related to calcitonin structurally — calcitonin gene-related peptide (CGRP), and islet amyloid polypeptide (IAPP); CGRP may be important in inducing relaxation of the smooth muscle in blood-vessel walls, and IAPP constitutes the amyloid which is found deposited in the islets of people with Type II diabetes. The physiological role of IAPP is not known, but it is normally secreted with insulin from the islets of Langerhans, and circulates (in minute amounts) in serum.

Osteomalacia and hypocalcaemia

The serum calcium concentration is normally tightly controlled. This is essential for normal depolarization of nerve and muscle cells. If there is a tendency to hypocalcaemia for any reason — dietary or metabolic — the body buffers the tendency by leaching calcium from the the large store in the bones. Parathyroid hormone is essential for this process. If the tendency persists for any length of time, the bones become thin and deformed. This is called osteomalacia. If PTH is missing, it is not possible to mobilize calcium from the bones and the person presents with hypocalcaemia rather than osteomalacia.

Factors tending to lower serum calcium concentration
A number of different factors may tend to lower serum calcium, and hence pre-dispose to the development of either hypocalcaemia or osteomalacia. In general terms they are the result of either calcium deficiency or vitamin D deficiency.

Calcium

Absorption
Dietary deficiency does not occur but there may be reduced absorption of calcium because of chelation in the gut. Phytates (as in high-cereal foods, e.g. chapattis) can do this. Calcium absorption is vitamin D-dependent and will be reduced by any cause of vitamin D deficiency.

Renal failure
In addition to the failure of 1α-hydroxylation of cholecalciferol, hypocalcaemia occurs because of phosphate retention.

Acute pancreatitis
Hypocalcaemia occurs due to the deposition of serum calcium as calcium phosphate and calcium soaps. In chronic pancreatitis there may be steattorhoea, with fat (and hence vitamin D) malabsorption.

Hypoparathyroidism
Any cause of PTH deficiency or PTH resistance may lead to hypocalcaemia.

Vitamin D

Dietary
Dietary causes are most common in the malnourished and deprived, and in those with fat malabsorption (vitamin D is a steroid and fat-soluble).

Reduced sunlight exposure
A tendency to dietary deficiency may become critical if there is associated reduced exposure to sunlight (ultraviolet light), with reduced production of cholecalciferol in the skin. This seems to be one reason why people of Indian origin in the UK are prone to osteomalacia. Nuclear submariners may be deprived of sunlight for months on end.

Renal
Defective 1α-hydroxylation of cholecalciferol in the kidney occurs in renal failure. Congenital absence of renal 1α-hydroxylase also occurs (very rarely).

Drugs
Anticonvulsants cause effective vitamin D deficiency – partly by an effect on the liver, and partly by inducing tissue resistance.

Tissue resistance
Tissue resistance can be acquired (anticonvulsant therapy, and diffuse gastro-intestinal disease) or inherited (vitamin D-resistant rickets, hypophosphataemic rickets).

Chronic liver disease
Osteomalacia can occur for mutiple reasons, including defective 25-hydroxylation of vitamin D and fat malabsorption.

Diffuse gastrointestinal disease
Coeliac disease and previous gastric surgery can lead to vitamin D deficiency.

Osteomalacia

Osteomalacia is the demineralization of bone resulting from calcium and/or vitamin D deficiency. The demineralization is the result of PTH acting on bone to maintain a normal serum calcium concentration.

Biochemical changes (Table 13.2)
Serum calcium will be low normal (rarely, frankly low) and serum PTH will be high (although it is not routinely measured). The urine calcium concentration will be low. The high PTH will leach calcium from the bone, and this results in secondary remodelling by osteoblasts. These osteoblasts release alkaline phosphatase into the blood. As a result of the calcium-conserving effect of PTH on the kidney, serum phosphate is low. Urinary cAMP is high.

Histological and radiological appearance of bone
Bones are demineralized, and are thin on X-ray. In childhood there are specific radiological abnormalities observable at the ends of growing long bones — widening of the epiphyseal plate and splaying of the diaphysis. This is called rickets. Widening of the ribs adjacent to the costal cartilage is the cause of the classic 'rickety rosary'. If untreated, the bones of the legs become irreversibly bowed and shortened.

In adults osteomalacia tends to present with localized lucencies (called Milkman fractures, or Looser zones), particularly in the pelvis or femur. They can be painful. There is associated generalized muscle weakness from the hypocalcaemic tendency.

Table 13.2. Biochemical features accompanying osteomalacia

Calcium	Low or low normal
Phosphate	Low or low normal
Alkaline phosphatase (bone)	High
PTH (if measured)	High
Urinary cAMP (if measured)	High

Histological exmination of bone reveals defective mineralization, with wide osteoid seams.

Renal osteodystrophy

People with renal failure tend to develop osteomalacia for two main reasons:
1 Defective hydroxylation of vitamin D by the kidney.
2 Phosphate retention by the glomerulus, casing hypocalcaemia.
Bone remodelling in renal failure is distinctive — rugger-jersey spine.

Hypocalcaemia

When the corrected serum calcium concentration is less than 2.20 mmol litre^{-1}, the person is said to be hypocalcaemic. This respresents an ionized calcium concentration of less than 1.2 mmol litre^{-1}. As almost half the circulating calcium is bound to serum albumin, the measured total calcium is very dependent on the albumin concentration. Albumin concentrations fall — especially during acute ill-health — and this will result in apparent hypocalcaemia. It is for this reason that it is essential to correct the measured calcium before making the diagnosis (see Table 13.1).

Symptoms

The symptoms of hypocalcaemia are paraesthesiae of the hands and around the mouth, associated with non-specific muscle weakness, gastrointestinal upset and malaise. The symptoms may be spontaneous or precipitated by emotional stress (hyperventilation causes a fall in ionized calcium by inducing respiratory alkalosis).

Signs

If a sphygmomanometer cuff around the arm is inflated above systolic pressure for 3 minutes, the muscles of the hand will go into painful carpopedal spasm — metacarpophalangeal flexion with extension of the interphalangeal joints (Trousseau's test). Tapping the cheek over the parotid gland may elicit a twitch of the facial muscles at the corner of the mouth (Chvostek's sign), but the sign is non-specific and of little use in clinical practice. On the ECG (electrocardiogram) there is prolongation of the Q–T interval. Papilloedema (caused by raised intracranial pressure) can occur in hypoparathyroidism.

When hypocalcaemia is gross, the person develops tetany. This is characterized by muscle contractions and cramps, associated with episodes of confusion, dizzy spells, collapses and fits. It can cause pulmonary oedema from left-ventricular failure. Hypocalcaemia in infancy and early childhood can cause irreversible mental retardation. There may be malformation of the teeth and nails.

Chronic hypocalcaemia is associated with steatorrhoea, intractable mucocutaneous moniliasis, cataracts and intracerebral calcification, but it is not completely clear whether these are the result of the hypocalcaemia or whether all are part of a multisystem disorder (see HAM syndrome, below).

Hypoparathyroidism

Hypoparathyroidism causes hypocalcaemia rather than osteomalacia.

Table 13.3. Causes of PTH deficiency

Hypoparathyroidism
Surgical, autoimmune, iatrogenic (see below)

Pseudohypoparathyroidism (PTH resistance)
Rare congenital syndromes (see below)

Magnesium depletion
Mg^{++} is a cofactor for some actions of PTH

Neonatal
Suppression of fetal parathyroid by maternal hypercalcaemia

Causes

The causes of deficient PTH activity are listed in Table 13.3. The commonest cause is surgery to the neck, either for hyperparathyroidism or for disease of the thyroid, pharynx and larynx. Congenital absence of the parathyroid glands is called the DiGeorge syndrome. Idiopathic hypoparathyroidism occurs, but is rare: the quoted prevalence of 1 in 5000 seems an overestimate. There are a number of familial syndromes, but hypoparathyroidism can also be sporadic.

In non-surgical acquired hypoparathyroidism the glands become underactive as a result of glandular atrophy. It may be autoimmune, and is often associated with other autoimmune glandular disease, and antiparathyroid antibodies have been demonstrated in a third of cases. The condition develops insidiously, most commonly in childhood and adolescence. Approximately 50% of cases form part of the HAM syndrome (hypoparathyroidism, Addison's disease, moniliasis — as well as pernicious anaemia), and any young person found to have Addison's disease should have hypoparathyroidism excluded. Hypoparathyroidism needs to be excluded also in any adult or child with non-specific symptoms of malaise, weakness and dizzy spells.

Clinical

The symptoms and signs are those of hypocalcaemia.

Diagnosis

The diagnosis is made by demonstrating signs of hypocalcaemia (low corrected serum calcium concentration), hyperphosphataemia (because PTH increases renal phosphate excretion), and an inappropriately low PTH concentration (because PTH should be high in the face of hypocalcaemia). There is reduced renal excretion of AMP.

Pseudohypoparathyroidism

This represents a group of inherited conditions with tissue resistance to PTH — they are usually X-linked dominant with variable penetrance. Affected people have a characteristic appearance: a short round face, short neck and short metacarpals. They have hypocalcaemia with high levels of PTH. There are different sorts of cellular defect which cause the tissue resistance. Treatment is as for hypopara-thyroidism.

Pseudopseudohypoparathyroidism is the name given to those who have the phenotype of pseudohypoparathyroidism, but in whom calcium metabolism is normal. It is a silly name, but nobody ever forgets it.

Treatment

Osteomalacia

Treatment rests on identifying and correcting the cause, and on the administration of vitamin D supplements. Small doses of oral vitamin D are sufficient: 400–500 U (10–12.5 µg) daily. This is available in tablets combined with calcium (Tabs Calcium and Vitamin D BPC) but the calcium is probably unnecessary.

In people with renal failure the main problem is one of defective hydroxylation of absorbed vitamin D. They are treated with 1 α-OH cholecalciferol (alfacalcidol) 1–2 µg daily. 1,25-OHCC (calcitriol) is also available but has no inherent advantage.

Hypoparathyroidism

It is not possible to correct the deficiency by giving PTH itself, and the aim of treatment is to compensate for lack of PTH by giving calcium and vitamin D to increase gastrointestinal absorption of calcium. Administration of vitamin D also compensates for the reduced renal hydroxylation of 25-OHCC which occurs in hypoparathyroidism.

Traditional treatment involves a combination of 1.0–1.5 g calcium with 0.25–20 mg (10 000–800 000 U) ergocalciferol (vitamin D_2). This regimen can cause problems because dose titration is difficult, and there can be wide swings from hypercalcaemia to hypocalcaemia.

Management is easier and safer with 1 α-OHCC (alfacalcidol) or 1,25-OHCC (calcitriol), in doses of 1–2 µg each day. Serum calcium should be measured frequently in the first few weeks of treatment, and subsequently each 6 months.

Emergency treatment of hypocalcaemia

Emergency treatment involves the intravenous administration of 10–30 ml of 10% calcium gluconate two to three times each day — by slow injection or by infusion in saline or 5% dextrose.

Hypercalcaemia

There are two common causes of hypercalcaemia, and many rare ones. A good working rule is that someone found to have mild hypercalcaemia will probably have primary hyperparathyroidism, and someone found to have severe hypercalcaemia will probably have a malignancy.

Definition

Serum calcium is said to be high when the corrected serum concentration is consistently greater than 2.60 mmol litre^{-1}. This represents an ionized concentration of greater than 1.45 mmol litre^{-1}.

Clinical

The symptoms and signs are vague and non-specific, and some people have none at all — even when the serum calcium concentration is very high. The diagnosis is usually made as a result of routine biochemical screening.

Those who do have symptoms may complain of malaise, depression, muscle weakness, anorexia, constipation, abdominal pain, polyuria (caused by hypercalcaemic damage to the renal tubule: nephrogenic diabetes insipidus) and, sometimes, renal colic from stones. The only signs which might be detected are corneal calcification (which resembles arcus senilis), and shortening of the Q–T interval on the electrocardiogram (ECG). X-rays may show renal calcification (nephrocalcinosis or stone formation).

Causes

The causes of hypercalcaemia are listed in Table 13.4. Note that secondary hyperparathyroidism is not associated with hypercalcaemia, but tertiary hyperparathyroidism is.

Differential diagnosis

If the hypercalcaemia is caused by hyperparathyroidism, serum phosphate will be lowish and urinary phosphate will be highish. Furthermore, urinary calcium will be proportionately low for the serum calcium because the action of PTH is to increase tubular reabsorption of calcium while increasing the excretion of phosphate. Various nomograms have been devised over the years: measures of renal tubular handling of phosphate or calcium. Note that samples for serum phosphate concentration need to be taken fasting, because of the amount of phosphate in food. Serum phosphate is of no help if the person has renal failure, because phosphate is retained when the glomeruli are damaged.

In severe hypercalcaemia it may be necessary to do a number of other tests to establish the cause. These include X-rays to detect radiological evidence of

Table 13.4. Causes of hypercalcaemia

Commoner causes
Primary hyperparathyroidism
Metastatic malignancy
Non-metastatic malignancy

Rarer causes
Tertiary hyperparathyroidism
Sarcoidosis
High bone turnover with immobilization (e.g. Paget's disease)
Vitamin D intoxication
Hyperthyroidism
Addison's disease
Thiazide diuretics
Hypercalcaemia of infancy
Familial benign hypercalcaemia
Milk-alkali syndrome (possibly)

---

hyperparathyroidism; tests to demonstrate malignancy — ESR, liver function tests, acid phosphatase (prostate), mammography (breast), skeletal survey or bone scan, chest X-ray, computed tomography (CT) scan, gastrointestinal imaging, tests for myeloma — ESR, immunoglobulin electrophoresis.

Primary hyperparathyroidism

Cause

Eighty per cent of cases are the result of an adenoma in a parathyroid gland, and 5% are the result of multiple adenomata. Carcinoma occurs in only 1% and there is usually little doubt about the diagnosis: the tumour is easily palpable and hard, and the serum PTH and calcium levels are very high. The remaining 10–15% are the result of hyperplasia of all four glands. This suggests that the glands are being stimulated by some other factor, but if they are, its identity is obscure.

Primary hyperparathyroidism is said to affect 0.1% of the population.

Clinical

The glands are rarely palpable and the symptoms — if any — are those of hypercalcaemia; 50% present with renal stone formation (but only 5%, or less, of people with renal colic have hyperparathyroidism). Excessive PTH secretion causes characteristic X-ray changes, but they are not present in everyone and probably reflect disease duration and severity (Table 13.5). With increased routine measurement of serum calcium, hyperparathyroidism is detected increasingly early, and bone changes are becoming a rarity.

Diagnosis

The diagnosis is suggested by hypercalcaemia in association with a low fasting serum phosphate. The finding of radiological evidence such as subperiosteal erosions is strongly suggestive. Isotope scans of the parathyroid are occasionally

Table 13.5. Radiological features of hyperparathyroidism

The radiological features are all the result of dissolution of bone by osteoclasts

Generalized osteopenia
Radiolucency, thin bones

Subperiosteal erosions
Small erosions especially seen at the margins of the phalanges and metacarpals

Pepperpot skull
Subperiosteal erosions in the calvarium

Loss of the lamina dura of the tooth sockets
There is no clear line between the roots of the teeth and the maxilla/mandible

Brown tumours
Sometimes the activated osteoclasts form macroscopic tumours — osteoclastomas. They are called 'brown tumours' because they are brown when cut across

---

helpful in localizing tumours; CT scans are rarely helpful because the overactive glands are not usually big enough to be seen. Serum PTH will be inappropriately elevated.

Treatment

There is only one effective treatment, and that is surgery. Most manage patients conservatively (i.e. do nothing except advise moderate restriction of calcium intake, but increase oral fluids to reduce urinary calcium concentration). There are, however, four relative indications for intervention:

1 Symptoms which are clearly related to the problem.
2 Evidence of hypercalcaemic renal damage.
3 Youth of the patient.
4 Severity of disease (e.g. corrected serum calcium > 3.00 mmol litre^{-1}).

In the rare situation in which primary hyperparathyroidism presents as an emergency with gross hypercalcaemia, it should be managed as described on p. 230.

Idiopathic hypercalciuria

Idiopathic hypercalciuria is the name given to the excessive urinary excretion of calcium (greater than approximately 6.00 mmol day^{-1}) in people with a normal serum calcium. As the serum phosphate is sometimes low, it has been suggested that idiopathic hypercalciuria may be a variant of hyperparathyroidism. This is not generally accepted, however. None the less, it is common, and is the commonest cause of renal stone formation.

Treatment

Treatment involves reducing dietary calcium and vitamin D, and increasing fluid intake. Reducing sodium intake also helps, as this increases sodium reabsorption in the proximal tubule and calcium is reabsorbed with it. Thiazide diuretics also increase calcium reabsorption (even though they increase sodium excretion). Finally, calcium absorption from the gut can be reduced with calcium binders such as cellulose phosphate.

Tertiary hyperparathyroidism

When there is a persistent tendency to hypocalcaemia — as in vitamin D deficiency or in renal failure — there is physiological hypertrophy of the parathyroid glands. This is called secondary hyperparathyroidism. When this stimulus is continued for so long that one or more of the glands becomes autonomous and overactive — even when the serum calcium starts to rise — this is called tertiary hyperparathyroidism.

The hyperparathyroidism (secondary or tertiary) of renal failure causes a typical X-ray appearance: rugger-jersey spine. In the days when sports colours were used more for team identity than as a source of income generation, it was traditional in the UK for players of rugby football to have horizontal stripes on their jerseys, whereas players of Association football had vertical ones. The namers of radiological signs missed the chance of giving the name 'soccer-shirt spine' to the vertical stripes seen in the vertebrae in osteoporosis (see p. 232).

Treatment

Treatment is as for primary hyperparathyroidism, but there is always a risk of recurrence if the underlying cause is uncorrected.

Hypercalcaemia of malignancy

Eighty per cent of cases investigated for hypercalcaemia in hospital will prove to have a malignancy. The tumours will be either those which commonly metastasize to bone (thyroid, breast, ovary, kidney, prostate), or those which do not (typically, tumours of the gastrointestinal tract and squamous tumours of the foregut and bronchus). Apart from these, myeloma is commonly associated with hyper-calcaemia.

If there are metastases in bone, they may cause bone dissolution and the release of calcium by the secretion of prostaglandins, cytokines or some other substance. When tumours cause hypercalcaemia without there being metastases present, it is by the release of humoral factors which induce bone resorption — osteoclast-activating factors, cytokines and parathyroid hormone-related protein (PTHrP).

Clinical

The hypercalcaemia tends to be severe and, in addition to the symptoms and signs listed above, the person may be markedly dehydrated from the polyuric effect of hypercalcaemia; they may be comatose, and can die.

Emergency treatment of hypercalcaemia

The urgent priority is to correct the dehydration with intravenous infusion of saline (with potassium, as indicated): up to 8 litres over 48 hours. Serum calcium concentration will fall only a little in response to rehydration, but the patient will feel a lot better.

Biphosphonates prevent calcium release from bone. They have to be given by infusion. Pamidronate is given as a single infusion of 30 mg, but can be repeated every 2–3 weeks. Other biphosphonates are etidronate and clodronate.

Calcitonin (25–100 U i.m. or s.c. three times daily) paralyses osteoclasts and reduces calcium for 2–3 days. It should be used if biphosphonates are ineffective. Plicamycin (mithramycin) also inhibits osteoclasts and acts for up to 10 days after a single infusion of 25 μg kg^{-1} over 4 hours.

Other treatments include peritoneal dialysis and oral phosphate (2–3 g day^{-1}). Steroids such as prednisolone are effective only in selected conditions, such as sarcoidosis, myeloma and lymphoma.

METABOLIC BONE DISEASE

Structure and function of bone

The main function of the skeleton is to support the body, but the bones also represent a large — and mobilizable — store of essential minerals, calcium and phosphate. The substance of bone is constantly remodelled, and the calcium and phosphate within it are in dynamic equilibrium with minerals in the extracellular space. The metabolism of bone is co-ordinated by three types of cell — osteoblasts, osteocytes and osteoclasts.

Osteoblasts

Osteoblasts are reticuloendothelial cells which are involved in laying down new bone (synthesizing mucopolysaccharides and collagen matrix), and in mineralizing it. They secrete alkaline phosphatase: an elevation of (bone) alkaline phosphatase in the blood indicates increased osteoblast activity.

Osteocytes

Osteocytes are derived from osteoblasts. They are found on the bone surface, or within lacunae. Osteocytes contribute to bone resorption (osteocytic osteolysis), but their detailed function is not known.

Osteoclasts

Osteoclasts are derived from haemopoietic precursors and aggregate into multi-nucleate giant cells. They are found on the surface of bone and their main function is bone resorption. Bone breakdown is essential for remodelling to occur, as well as to enable the release of calcium and phosphate at times of need.

Metabolic diseases of bone

There are many different disorders of bone, both congenital and acquired. The only ones which are considered here are the common ones — the ones which relate to disorders of calcium metabolism, and the ones which are referred to endocrinologists for management. One rare exception which should be mentioned is the congenital disorder, the McCune–Albright syndrome (see p. 191). Affected children (usually girls) have polyostotic fibrous dysplasia (multiple fractures from defective bone formation), with geographical pigmentation of the skin (brown blotches like countries on a map of the world) and precocious puberty and, sometimes, tumours of the pituitary gland.

Osteomalacia

Osteomalacia is the disorder of bone which results from lack of calcium or vitamin D. There is defective mineralization of new osteoid, as well as increased extraction of calcium from bone by PTH in an attempt to maintain normocalcaemia. This is discussed in detail above.

Hyperparathyroidism

Parathyroid hormone stimulates osteoclastic resorption of bone. Bones are generally thinned, but there are characteristic radiological abnormalities' (see Table 13.5).

Osteoporosis

In osteoporosis there is loss of the protein matrix of bone. This contrasts with osteomalacia, in which the protein structure of bone is normal (more or less) but poorly calcified. Osteoporosis is a common feature of ageing, and hence it is possible to argue that the osteoporotic thinning of the bones in old age is 'normal'. When thinning is so marked that the bones become compressed (e.g. vertebrae) or fractured (e.g. neck of femur), there is little doubt that the process is abnormal.

Causes

Not much is known of the control of the formation of the collagen structure of bone. However, it reaches its peak in mature adulthood, and the height of the peak determines the relative risk of bones becoming abnormally thin later. The peak bone mass is determined by race (Blacks have more) and by sex (males have more). It is also determined by overall body weight and physical activity (the fatter and the fitter have more). The high oestrogens of pregnancy also increase bone mass, and multiparae are less likely to develop osteoporosis in later life than women who are childless. Long-term use of oestrogen-containing contraceptives may also have a protective effect. Once bone mass has achieved its peak it begins to decline inexorably with advancing age, and the rate of decline is greatest in women after the menopause. Hormone replacement therapy (HRT) reduces this decline, but will not replace bone which has already been lost.

It follows that women (and especially White women), who are most at risk, can reduce the chances of developing problems by either being plump people who take regular physical exercise as youngish adults, and/or by taking HRT from the time of the menopause. The reason why oestrogens protect the skeleton of women is not known for certain. However, oestrogens increase GH secretion by the pituitary and may increase IGF_1 activity in bone.

Androgens also protect the skeleton: men with long-standing hypogonadism can develop osteoporosis.

Other factors

Other causes of generalized osteoporosis include excessive steroid therapy (or Cushing's syndrome), thyrotoxicosis and excessive alcohol intake.

Clinical

The symptoms are those of pain, deformity and fracture. The pain from osteoporotic collapse of vertebrae may be felt in the back, or referred to dermatomes because of compression of the dorsal roots. Back pain can be very severe, but tends to improve after 2–3 months.

The fractures (especially of the ribs) of people with Cushing's are usually painless, and those of alcoholism are usually unremembered.

The appearances on X-ray are characteristic: generalized thinning, especially of the cortex, fractures in sites of stress (neck of femur, vertebrae), increased prominence of vertical trabeculae of the vertebrae giving vertical stripes, and indentation of the vertebrae ('codfish spine'). Loss of vertical height occurs as a result of vertebral compression, and kyphosis (forward bending) occurs from wedge fractures.

Treatment

There is no proven treatment for established osteoporosis. Prevention with HRT is the only logical strategy. Calcium and vitamin D administration probably play no useful part in either prevention or treatment — it is collagen which is deficient, not calcium.

The use of sodium fluoride (NaF) may be indicated in some cases. This stabilizes the bone and makes it resistant to dissolution. It may increase bone mass. Gastrointestinal side-effects are common.

Paget's disease of bone

Paget's disease of bone is a disease of osteoclasts, and is probably caused by a slow virus. Racial susceptibility is important — Anglo-Saxons seem to be prone to it whereas other Caucasians are not. It is rare, for instance, in Scandinavia, but affects 3–4% of the population in the UK, particularly in northern industrial towns. It is common in countries colonized by Anglo-Saxons: the USA and Australasia. It is commoner in men than women, and commoner with advancing age.

Pathology

Excessive activity of the osteoclasts causes excessive bone resorption. Calcium and collagen breakdown products (hydroxyproline) escape into the blood, and are thence excreted in the urine. If an affected person is immobilized for any reason, there may be transient hypercalcaemia because of an increase in bone breakdown.

Osteoblasts struggle to correct the problem by laying down new bone. Serum alkaline phosphatase concentrations are very high as a result. However, the osteoclasts do not remodel the new bone and it is misshapen, expanded, poorly calcified, soft and compressible (vertebrae), or bendable (weight-bearing long bones). It is vascular, and the overlying skin may be warm. It is often painful — presumably due to stimulation of the pain fibre terminals in the stretched periosteum.

Clinical

Ninety-five per cent of cases are asymptomatic, and the diagnosis is made by chance (alkaline phosphatase elevated, incidental finding on X-ray). Otherwise the symptoms and signs are pain (constant, aching, drawing pain in the affected bone), deformity, and the results of compression of adjacent structures (e.g. spinal cord, cranial nerves) by expanded bone. Heart failure can occur because of increased cardiac output. Osteosarcoma is a rare (1%) complication.

Diagnosis

The X-ray appearances are diagnostic. Alkaline phosphatase is high in the serum. Urinary hydroxyproline is high, and is a good marker of the activity of osteoclasts.

Treatment

The structure of bone can be made resistant to the action of osteoclasts by giving biphosphonates such as pamidronate or etidronate. Alternatively, osteoclasts can be inhibited by giving calcitonin by subcutaneous injection (usually 100 U three times weekly). Plicamycin (mithramycin) also inhibits osteoclasts, but is toxic to the bone marrow.

In general terms, treatment should only be given for symptoms. Those without major problems should be left alone, or managed with simple analgesia.

Index

Page numbers in *italics* indicate tables or figures.

ACE *85*, 86, *87*
Acne 83, 95, 210
Acromegaly 53–5, 119
Acropachy 66, 71
ACTH *see* Adrenocorticotrophic hormone
Activin 40, 194
Addisonian crisis 92, 93
Addison's disease 83, 84, 91–2, 225
 causes 90
Adenocarcinoma, renal 103, 108
Adenomas
 adrenal 96, 100, 101
 parathyroid 228
 pituitary *see* Pituitary tumours
 thyroid 65, 68, *70*
Adenylate cyclase 22–3, 24
ADH *see* Antidiuretic hormone
Adipocytes
 metabolism 166
 regional variation 166
 response to obesity and fasting 167
 size and number 166–7
 T_3 and 167
Adipose tissue, brown (BAT) 167
Adrenal adenomas 96, 100, 101
Adrenal carcinoma 96, 99, 100
Adrenal cortex
 adrenal medulla interactions 7–8, 79
 control of function 84
 diseases 89–101
 hormones 15–17, 80–4
 kidney interactions 79, *85*
 structure 79, *81*
Adrenalectomy 53, 99, 101
Adrenal gland 79–80
Adrenal hyperplasia 52, 96, 100
 congenital *see* Congenital adrenal hyperplasia
Adrenaline 6–9, 79, 84
 secretion 8, 80
 target cell interactions 8, 24
Adrenal medulla
 adrenal cortex interactions 7–8, 79
 diseases 103–6
 hormones 7–8, 84
 structure 79–80, *81*
α-Adrenoceptors *8*, 24
β-Adrenoceptors *8*, 24
Adrenocortical failure 89–92, 115
Adrenocorticotrophic hormone (ACTH) 36–7, 79
 control of adrenal cortex function 84
 deficiency 30, 44–6, 57, *58*, *90*, 91
 ectopic secretion *see* Ectopic ACTH syndrome
 plasma concentrations 52, 91, 95, 98–9

 -secreting pituitary tumours 41, 51–3, 96, 98, 99
 secretion 3, *26*, 33, *34*, 36–7
Adrenocorticotrophic hormone-related
  peptides 36–7
Adrenoleukodystrophy 90, 91
Adrenomyeloneuropathy 90, 91
Age
 bone 184, *185*, 192
 heart disease risk and 163
 lipoprotein metabolism and 156–7
 male sexual function and 194
AI *see* Artificial insemination
Albumin
 calcium binding 220, 224
 thyroid hormone binding 12–13, 63
 urinary excretion 141
Alcohol (ethanol)
 flushing attacks 119
 hypoglycaemic effects 115, 135
 impotence and 197
 lipoprotein metabolism and 156, 158, 161
Alcohol (ethanol) abuse
 hypertension 89
 osteoporosis 232
 pseudo-Cushing's syndrome 96–7
Aldose reductase *139*
Aldosterone *16*, 44–5, 80, 82–3
 actions 82–3, *87*, 88
 control of secretion 84, *85*, 86, 88
 deficiency 83, 95
 see also Addison's disease; Hyperaldosteronism
Alfacalcidol (1α-OH cholecalciferol) 102, 226
Alkaline phosphatase 223, 231, 233
Amenorrhoea 28, 211
 secondary 48, 213–14
 see also Puberty, delayed
AMH *see* Antimullerian hormone
Aminoglutethimide 53, *90*, 100
Amphetamine derivatives 171
Amputations, diabetes 148, 149
Amylin (islet amyloid polypeptide) 125, 221
Amyotrophy, diabetic 145
Anabolic steroids 189–90, 212
Androgens 40, 204
 adrenal 83, 187
 congenital adrenal hyperplasia 94, 95
 Cushing's syndrome 98
 deficiency 199, 200–1, 202
 excess 83, 178, 211–12, 213
 growth and 186
 osteoporosis and 232
 polycystic ovary syndrome 210
 resistance 178–9, 202
 sexual differentiation and 174–5, *176*
 treatment 212
 tumours secreting 83, 178, 201, 202, 209, 211

see also Testosterone; other specific androgens
Andrology   193–203
Androstenedione   16, 83, 94
Aneurysms   28, 42
ANF see Atrial natriuretic factor
Angiotensin-converting enzyme (ACE)   85, 86, 87
Angiotensin II (AII)   84, 85, 86, 88
Anion exchange resins   165
Ankle swelling   98
Anorchia   179–80
Anorexia nervosa   172, 213
   hyperlipidaemia   159, 160
   hypothalamic dysfunction   28, 51, 172
Anovulation   213–14, 215
Antiandrogens   192, 196, 213
Anticonvulsants   222
Antidiuretic hormone (ADH, AVP)   26, 27
   actions   87, 88
   deficiency   29, 44
   syndrome of inappropriate secretion
      (SIADH)   32–3
   tumours secreting   108
Antimullerian hormone (AMH, MIF)   173, 172,
      176, 177
Antioestrogens   202
Antithyroglobulin antibodies   65, 66, 77
Antithyroid drugs   71–3, 72–4
Anxiety, flushing attacks   118
Apoprotein CII (apo CII) deficiency   161
Apoproteins   154, 155
Appetite, CNS control   169
Appetite-suppressant drugs   171
Arachidonic acid derivatives   17–19, 23, 152
Arginine, intravenous   184
Arginine vasopressin see Antidiuretic hormone
Arteriosclerosis, pathogenesis   162–3
Artificial insemination (AI)   50, 200, 215
Asian patients, diabetes mellitus   130–1
Atherosclerosis   140, 162–3
Atrial natriuretic factor (ANF, atriopeptin)   87–8
Autocrine actions   1
Autoimmune disease
   Addison's disease   90
   diabetes mellitus   124, 125
   hypoparathyroidism   225
   pregnancy and   218
   thyroid gland   65–7
Autonomic neuropathy, diabetic   119, 141, 146–7,
      148
AVP see Antidiuretic hormone
Azoospermia   198, 199, 200

Baldness, male pattern   83, 98
Bartter's syndrome   103
Basal metabolic rate (BMR), obesity   167–8
BAT see Adipose tissue, brown
Behaviour modification
   anorexia nervosa   172
   obesity   170–1
Biphosphonates   230, 233
α-Blockers   105
β-Blockers
   adverse effects   125, 158, 161, 196
   phaeochromocytoma   105
   thyrotoxicosis   73, 74

Blood pressure, raised see Hypertension
BMI see Body mass index
BMR see Basal metabolic rate
Body-builders   202, 203
Body mass index (BMI)   165
Bombesin   110, 111
Bone   230–3
   mass   232
   metabolic diseases   231–3
   metastases   230
   structure and function   230–1
Bone age   184, 185, 192
Bradykinin   86
Brain, complications of diabetes   138, 139–40
Breast
   enlargement, boys   187, 194, 202
   progesterone actions   206
Breastfeeding, antithyroid drugs and   75
Breast tumours   107
Bromocriptine   52, 54–5, 56, 57, 102
Bronchial carcinoma see Lung carcinoma
Bronchospasm   19
Brown adipose tissue (BAT)   167
Brown tumours, hyperparathyroidism   228
Bulimia   172
Bulking agents   171

Caffeine (coffee)   158, 169
CAH see Congenital adrenal hyperplasia
Calcitonin   221
   treatment   221, 230, 233
   tumours secreting   69, 106
Calcitonin gene-related peptide (CGRP)   221
Calcitriol see 1,25-Dihydroxycholecalciferol
Calcium
   absorption   219, 222
   deficiency   222
   homeostasis   219–20
   intracellular   23–4
   metabolism   102, 219–130
   serum   223, 226, 227
      factors lowering   222–3
      total corrected   220
   treatment   226
   urinary   223
Calmodulin   23–4
Candidiasis, vaginal   122
Carbimazole   71–3, 74, 75
Carbohydrates, dietary intake   157
Carcinoid syndrome   117–18, 119
Carcinoid tumours   116–18, 120
Cardiomyopathy, diabetes mellitus   140
Cardiovascular risk factors   162–3
Carpal tunnel syndrome   144
Cataracts   143
Catecholamines   4, 6–9, 84, 87
   hypoglycaemic symptoms and   115
   inactivation and clearance   8–9
   plasma/urinary concentrations   104
   secretion   8
   synthesis   7–8
   target-cell interaction   8
   see also Adrenaline; Noradrenaline
Catechol-O-methyl transferase (COMT)   8–9
CBG see Cortisol-binding globulin

C-cells (parafollicular cells), thyroid 221
CCK *see* Cholecystokinin
Cellulitis 148
Cervical mucus 215
CGRP *see* Calcitonin gene-related peptide
Charcot foot 149
CHD *see* Coronary heart disease
Cheiroarthropathy, diabetic 142–3
Chemotherapy, cancer 108
Children
 growth 181
 luteinizing hormone and follicle-stimulating
  hormone deficiency 48
 small stature 28, 47, 182–6, 190
 tall stature 186–7
Chlorpropamide 31, 132, 133
Cholecalciferol (vitamin D$_3$) 14, 220
Cholecystokinin (CCK) 109, 110
Cholesterol 152
 metabolism 152–4
 serum
  atherosclerosis and 162
  factors affecting 156–7
  heart disease risk 162
 steroid hormones derived from 13–17
Cholestyramine 165
Chorioncarcinoma 75, 108, 201
Chorionic gonadotrophin, human (hCG) 217
 stimulation test 189
 structure 3, 5, 39
 testicular development and 179, 180, 193–4
 thyroid stimulation 63, 74, 75, 218
 treatment 50, 51, 189, 190, 200, 216
 tumours secreting 108, *191*, 201
Chromaffin cells 80
Chromogranin A 80
Chromosomal abnormalities 177–8, 191
Chromosomes, sex 173
Chvostek's sign 224
Chylomicrons 154, *156*
Cimetidine 196
Circadian rhythms 19
Climacteric *see* Menopause
CLIP *see* Corticotrophin-like intermediate lobe
  peptide
Clitoromegaly 83, 94
Clofibrate 164
Clomiphene
 test 189, 190
 treatment 211, 216
Clonidine, oral 184
Clotting 18–19
Coeliac disease 223
Coffee (caffeine) 158, 169
Coital problems 214
Colestipol 165
Coma
 hyperosmolar non-ketotic 128
 myxoedema 77–8
Computed tomography (CT) scans 99, 105, 192
COMT *see* Catechol-O-methyl transferase
Condom devices, semi-rigid 198
Congenital adrenal hyperplasia (CAH) 83, 92–6,
  178
 clinical features 50, 93–4, 186, 212
 diagnosis 95

inheritance 93
 non-classical 94–5
 treatment 95–6
Conn's syndrome 89, 100–1
Corneal arcus 161
Coronary heart disease (CHD)
 diabetes mellitus 140
 risk factors *161*, 162–3
Corpus luteum 204, 206, 207, 216–17
Corticosteroids 15–17, 80–4
 replacement therapy 46, 92, *93*, 95–6
 synthesis 15, *16*
 treatment 211, 216, 230, 232
 see also Glucocorticoids; Mineralocorticoids;
  specific steroids
Corticosterone *16*, 80
Corticotrophin-like intermediate lobe peptide
  (CLIP) 36
Corticotrophin-releasing hormone (CRH) 36–7, 84
 deficiency 29
 test 52, 99
Cortisol (hydrocortisone) *16*, 21, 80
 catecholamine synthesis and 7–8
 deficiency 44–6, *83*, 89–92, 95
 plasma concentrations 45, *58*, 91
 treatment
  adrenocorticotrophic hormone cortisol
   deficiency 46, 57, 92, *93*, 95–6
  thyroid disease 74, 78
 24-hour urine excretion 52, 98, 169
Cortisol-binding globulin (CBG) 15
Cortisone acetate *93*
Cosmetic surgery
 gynaecomastia 202
 intersex states 179
 obesity 172
Cosmetic treatment, hirsutism 212
C-peptide 3, 4
Cramps, night 122
Cranial irradiation 108
Cranial nerve palsies 35–6, 43, 146
Craniopharyngioma 27–8
Cretinism 75, 77
Creutzfeld–Jakob disease 47, 186
CRH *see* Corticotrophin-releasing hormone
Cryptorchidism 179–80
CT scans *see* Computed tomography scans
Cushing's disease 51–3, 79, 96
 intermittent or cyclic 96
Cushing's syndrome 51, 81, 96–100, 107
 causes 96–7
 clinical features *82*, 89, 97–8, 168–9, 212, 232
 diagnosis 98–9
 diagnosis of cause 99
 treatment 99–100
Cyclic AMP 8, 22–3
 urinary 223
Cyclosporin 158
Cyproheptadine 52
Cyproterone acetate 192, 196, 213
Cytokines 21, 230
Cytology, fine-needle aspiration 65

DBP *see* Vitamin D-binding protein
DDAVP (deamino-D-arg-vasopressin) 31

Death, sudden   146
Decidua   217
Dehydroepiandrosterone (DHEA)   *16*, 94, 217
Dehydroepiandrosterone sulphate (DHEAS)   83, 217
Demeclocycline   33
Depression
   polycystic ovary syndrome   210
   post-partum   218
De Quervain's disease (subacute thyroiditis)   67, 76
Development   178–92
Dexamethasone   *93*
   suppression tests   52, 98, 99, 169
Dexfenfluramine   171
DG *see* Diacylglycerol
DHEA *see* Dehydroepiandrosterone
DHEAS *see* Dehydroepiandrosterane sulphate
DHT *see* Dihydrotestosterone
DI *see* Diabetes insipidus
Diabetes insipidus (DI)   28, 29–31
   cranial   29, 30, 31, 42, 44
   nephrogenic   29, 30, 31, 102
Diabetes mellitus (DM)   113, 121–48
   assessment of recently diagnosed   126
   'brittle'   137–8
   complications   137–49
   diagnosis   121–2
   dietary modification   131
   gestational   *123*, 125, 130
   hyperlipidaemia   156, 159, 160, 161
   hypoglycaemia   115, 132, 135–7, 141
   impotence   142, 146, 147, 196–7
   insulin treatment   133–7
   management   127–31
   management objectives   150
   maturity-onset, of young people (MODY)   125
   oral hypoglycaemic drug therapy   131–3
   pancreatic diseases   *123*, 125–6
   screening for complications   149–50
   secondary   54, 98, *123*
   type I (insulin-dependent)   102, 113, 123–4, 137
      diagnosis   126
      initial management   128–9
      insulin treatment   133–7
   type II (non-insulin-dependent)   113, *123*, 124–5, 137
      diagnosis   126
      initial management   130
      obesity   125, 168
      tablet treatment   131–3
   types   122–6
Diabetic autonomic neuropathy   119, 141, 146–7, *148*
Diabetic ketoacidosis   113, 123, 127
Diabetic nephropathy   *138*, 140–1
Diabetic neuropathies   *138*, 141, 142, 144–7
Diabetic retinopathy   141, 143–4
Diacylglycerol (DG)   23, 152
Diazoxide   114
DIDMOAD syndrome   30, 102
Diet
   calcium deficiency and   222
   diabetes mellitus and   125, 131, 133
   flushing and   118
   hirsutism and   212
   hyperlipoproteinaemia and   157–8, 164

   vitamin D deficiency   222
   weight-losing   170
Diethylpropion   171
Differentiation   173–80
Diffuse idiopathic skeletal hyperostosis (DISH)   143
DiGeorge syndrome   225
Digoxin   196
Dihydrotestosterone (DHT)   17, 174, *177*, 178
1,25-Dihydroxycholecalciferol (1,25-OHCC, calcitriol)   15, 219, 220
   synthesis   14
   treatment   102, 226
24,25-Dihydroxycholecalciferol (24,25-OHCC)   *14*, 15, 220
Diiodotyrosine (DIT)   *11*, 12, 62
DISH *see* Diffuse idiopathic skeletal hyperostosis
Dizziness   122, 146
DM *see* Diabetes mellitus
Dopamine   6–9, 84
   deficiency   29
   prolactin inhibition   19, 26, 38
Dopamine-receptor agonists   56, 57
Down-regulation, receptor   5–6, 22
Down's syndrome   76
Driving, diabetes mellitus   128, 136
Drug-induced disorders
   adrenocortical deficiency   *90*
   diabetes mellitus   114, 125
   flushing   119
   hirsutism   212
   hyperlipidaemia   158, 161
   hypocalcaemia   222
   impotence   196, *197*
   weight gain   169
Dwarfism, Laron-type   184

ECG *see* Electrocardiogram
Ectopic adrenocorticotrophic hormone syndrome   69, 96, 107, 116–17
   clinical features   98
   diagnosis   99
Ectopic hormone secretion   107
Education, hyperlipoproteinaemia   164
Ejaculation   198
Elderly, idiopathic hypopituitarism   29
Electrocardiogram (ECG)   224, 227
Electrolyte balance   *87*, 88
Emotional deprivation, childhood   183
Endocrine actions   1, 109
Endocrine system   1–24
Endometrial carcinoma   211
β-Endorphin   36
Enkephalins   79, 84
Enteroglucagon   *110*, 111
Enteroinsular axis hormones   109–19
Epinephrine *see* Adrenaline
Epiphyses   180, 181, *182*
EPO *see* Erythropoietin
Erection   195–8
Ergocalciferol (vitamin D$_2$)   14–15, 220, 226
Erythropoietin (EPO)   85, 88
   deficiency   102
   tumours secreting   103, 105, 108
Ethanol *see* Alcohol
Ethinyloestradiol   185, 190

Ethnic minorities, diabetes   130–1
Etomidate   *90*, 100
Eunuchoid stature   48, *49*, 54, 177, 186, 199
Exercise
    blood sampling after   184
    lipoprotein metabolism and   156, 157
    obesity and   170
    osteoporosis and   232
Eye
    diabetic autonomic neuropathy and   146
    screening in diabetes   149
Eye disease
    diabetes mellitus   *138*, 143–4
    thyroid   66, 71 *72*

Familial syndromes   105
Fanconi's syndrome   103
Fasting, adipocyte responses   167
Fat   151–72
    dietary intake   157
    malabsorption   222
    metabolism   151–72
Fatty acids
    free (FFA)   151, 152, 166
    saturated   157
Feeding, CNS control   169
Females
    genital tract abnormalities   215
    infertility   50–1, 190, 210, 211, 214–16
    luteinizing hormone and follicle-stimulating
        hormone deficiency   48, 50–1
    sexual differentiation   173–5
    sexual function   204–18
Feminization   *176*, 201
    testicular   178
Fenfluramine   171
Fetoplacental hormones   217
Fetus, growth   180
FFA *see* Fatty acids, free
FH *see* Hypercholesterolaemia, familial
Fibrates   164
Fibre, dietary   158
Fish oils   164–5
Fludrocortisone   46, 92, *93*
5-Fluorouracil   113, 114
Fluoxymesterone   189–90
Flushing attacks   118–19
Follicle-stimulating hormone (FSH)   39–41
    deficiency   44, 47–51, *58*, 200, 213
    female sexual function and   205, 206, 207
    gonadal failure   190
    menopausal women   207
    polycystic ovary syndrome   210
    puberty   187
    secretion   26, 33, *34*, 40–1
    structure   3, *5*, 39
    testicular function and   194
    treatment   50–1, 190, 200
    tumours secreting   41
Foot
    Charcot   149
    diabetic autonomic neuropathy   146–7
    drop   144
    ischaemic   140, 147–8
    neuroischaemic   148

    neuropathic   147
    problems in diabetes   *138*, 147–9
    screening in diabetes   149–50
Forrestier's disease   143
Fractures, spontaneous   98, 232
Frozen shoulder   143
FSH *see* Follicle-stimulating hormone

Galactorrhoea   57, 210, 211
    normoprolactinaemic   56–7
Ganglioneuroblastoma   113
Ganglioneuroma   104
Gangrene, diabetic foot   147, 148
Gastric bypass surgery   171–2
Gastric inhibitory peptide (GIP)   109, 110
Gastric plication (gastroplasty)   172
Gastrin   109–10
Gastrinoma   105, 109–10, 114
Gastrointestinal disease   223
Gastroparesis   146
Genitalia
    external   174, *177*
    internal   174, *175*
Germ-cell tumours, testes   201
Gestational diabetes   *123*, 125, 130
GH *see* Growth hormone
GHRH *see* Growth hormone-releasing hormone
GHRIH *see* Somatostatin
Gigantism (giantism)   53–5, 187
GIP *see* Gastric inhibitory peptide; Glucose-
    dependent insulinotropic peptide
Glibenclamide   132, 133
Gliclazide   132, 133
Glicentin   111
Glomerular hyperfiltration, diabetes mellitus
    140–1
Glomerulosclerosis, diabetes mellitus   140–1
Glucagon   109, *110*, 111, 112
    growth hormone responses   184
    treatment   136
Glucagonoma   113, 126
Glucocorticoids   79, 80, 81, 156
    actions   81, *82*
    control of secretion   84
    deficiency   44–6, *83*, 89–92, 95
    equivalent doses   *93*
    excess *see* Cushing's disease; Cushing's syndrome
    hypertensive effects   89, 98
    inactivation and clearance   17
    replacement therapy   46, 92, *93*, 95–6
    synthesis   *16*
    see also Cortisol
Glucose, blood
    concentrations   116, 121, 126
    problems of control in diabetes   137
Glucose-dependent insulinotrophic peptide
    (GIP)   109, 110
Glucose tolerance
    impaired (IGT)   122
    test   54, 122
Glycoprotein family of hormones   3, *5*, 39
Glycosuria   126
Glycosylation, non-enzymatic   139
GnRH *see* Gonadotrophin-releasing hormone
Goitre   67–9, 71

dyshormonogenetic 65, 68
endemic (iodine deficiency) 60, 67
multinodular 68, *70*
simple 67
Gonadal steroids 15–17
see also Sex steroids
Gonadotrophin-releasing hormone (GnRH) 26,
    39–40, 47
deficiency 29, 189, 190, 199, 200, 213
test 48, *58*, 189, 190, 192
treatment 180, 189, 192, 200, 216
Gonadotrophins
deficiency 44, 47–51, 200
female infertility 50–1, 190, 216
male infertility 50, *51*, 190, 200
see also Chorionic gonadotrophin, human; Follicle-
    stimulating hormone; Luteinizing hormone
Gonads
development 173–4
diabetes mellitus *138*, 141
irradiation 108
Gout 159
G-proteins 22–3
Granuloma annulare 142
Granulosa cells 204–5
Graves' disease 47, 69, 71
diagnosis 65, *70*, 71
goitre 67
pathogenesis 65–7
in pregnancy 74–5, 218
prognosis 73
see also Thyrotoxicosis
Graves' ophthalmopathy 66, 71, *72*
GRH *see* Growth hormone-releasing hormone
Growth *50*, 180–92
childhood 181
congenital adrenal hyperplasia *50*, 94
precocious puberty 192
spurt, puberty 181, *182*, *183*, 187
Tanner staging 187, *188*
velocity *181*, 184
Growth factors 180–1
Growth hormone (GH) 38
actions *37*, 38
deficiency 29, 46–7, 180, 182, 183–4
    pituitary tumours 44
    treatment 47, 185
growth and 80–1, *182*, *183*, 186, 187
reserve, biochemical assessment *58*, 184–5
resistance 184
-secreting pituitary tumours 41, 53–5, 57, 187
secretion 3–4, 19–20, 26, 33, *34*, 38
serum concentrations 54, 102, 185
therapy 47, 185–6
Growth hormone release-inhibiting hormone
    (GHRIH) *see* Somatostatin
Growth hormone-releasing hormone (GHRH,
    GRH) 20, 26, 38
deficiency 29, 183–4
test 185
Growth plate 180, 181, *182*
Gustatory sweating 119, 146
Gut hormones 109–19
Gynaecological endocrinology 204–18
Gynaecomastia 83, 177, 190, 202–3
causes 202

investigations 202–3
puberty 187, 194, 202

H_2 receptor antagonists 114
Haemangioblastomas 103, 105
Haemangiopericytomas, renal 103
Haemochromatosis 28, 90, 126
HAM syndrome 90, 225
Hashimoto's thyroiditis 66, 69, 76
diagnosis *70*, 77
goitre 67
hCG *see* Chorionic gonadotrophin, human
HDL *see* High-density lipoproteins
Headache, pituitary tumours 45
Head injury 28
Heart disease
coronary *see* Coronary heart disease
diabetes *138*, 140
Heart, vagal denervation 146
Heel ulcers 149
Height
loss of 232
velocity *181*, 184
Hepatic lipase 156, 160
Hermaphroditism, true 174, 176
High-density lipoproteins (HDL) *153*, 154, 156
factors affecting 157, 158, 159
reduced, heart disease risk 163
Hirsutism 83, 211–13
congenital adrenal hyperplasia 95
Cushing's syndrome 98
ovarian tumours 209
polycystic ovary syndrome 210
HLA haplotypes 65, 124
HMG *see* Human menopausal gonadotrophin
Homosexuality 175
Hormone replacement therapy (HRT) 50, 158,
    208, 209, 232
Hormones 1–24
control of secretion 19–21
ectopic secretion 107
factors modifying action 19–22
production by tumours 108
second messengers 22–4
tumour dependence 107
types 1–19
see also specific hormones
Hormone-sensitive lipase (HSL) 166
Hot flushes 41, 118, 207
HPL *see* Human placental lactogen
HRT *see* Hormone replacement therapy
HSL *see* Hormone-sensitive lipase
Human chorionic gonadotrophin *see* Chorionic
    gonadotrophin, human
Human menopausal gonadotrophin (HMG) 50, *51*,
    216
Human menopausal gonadotrophin Co-A
    reductase 152, 156
inhibitors 165
Human placental lactogen (HPL) 217
H–Y antigen 173
Hydatidiform moles 75, 108
Hydrocortisone *see* Cortisol
1α-Hydroxycholecalciferol (1α-OHCC,
    alfacalcidol) 102, 226

25-Hydroxycholecalciferol (25-OHCC)   *14*, 15
5-Hydroxyindoleacetic acid (5HIAA)   118
1α-Hydroxylase deficiency   222
21-Hydroxylase deficiency   93
17-Hydroxyprogesterone (17-OH
    progesterone)   *16*, 94, 95, 212
Hydroxyproline, urinary   233
5-Hydroxytryptamine (5-HT)   9–10, 116, 117–18
H–Y gene   173, 174
Hyperaldosteronism   83
    primary   89, 100–1
    secondary   *101*, 103
Hypercalcaemia   226–8
    adrenocortical failure   92
    of malignancy   107, 230
    treatment   221, 230
Hypercalciuria, idiopathic   229
Hypercholesterolaemia
    common (polygenic)   *161*
    drug therapy   165
    familial (FH)   156, 160, *161*
Hyperchylomicronaemia   *161*
Hyperemesis gravidarum   75, 218
Hyperglycaemia
    emergency management   127–8
    symptoms   *122*
Hyperinsulinaemia   89, 102, 112–13, 115
Hyperkalaemia   91
Hyperlipidaemia (hyperlipoproteinaemia)   156–61
    classification   160–61
    clinical manifestations   161
    factors causing   156–9
    familial combined   160, *161*
    management   163–5
    remnant   *161*
    secondary   158–9
Hyperosmolar non-ketotic coma (HONK)   128
Hyperostosis, diffuse idiopathic skeletal
        (DISH)   143
Hyperparathyroidism   231
    primary   105, 228–9
    secondary   102, 227
    tertiary   227, 229
Hyperphosphataemia   225
Hyperprolactinaemia   55–6, 57, 190
    causes   29, 41, 102
    clinical features   55–6, 168, 212, 213
    polycystic ovary syndrome   210, 211
Hypertension   89
    acromegaly   53
    atherosclerosis and   162
    Conn's syndrome   89, 100
    Cushing's sydnrome   89, 98
    diabetes mellitus   *138*, 140, 149
    heart disease risk and   163
    phaeochromocytoma   89, 104
    renal failure   102
    renovascular   89, 102
Hyperthyroidism *see* Thyrotoxicosis
Hypertriglyceridaemia
    drug therapy   164–5
    familial   *161*
    heart disease risk   163
Hypoadrenal (Addisonian) crisis   92, 93
Hypocalcaemia   102, 221–6
    diagnosis   224

emergency treatment   226
hypoparathyrodism   224–5
pseudohypoparathyroidism   225–6
Hypocortisolism   44–6, *83*, 89–92, 95
Hypoglycaemia   115–16
    causes   113, 114, 115–16
    clinical features   115, 119
    diabetes mellitus   115, 132, 135–7, 141
    diagnosis   116
    reactive   115–16
    tumour-associated   116
    unawareness   136–7
Hypoglycaemia stress (insulin tolerance) test   45,
        52, 98, 184
Hypogonadism   190
    gigantism and   53, 54
    hyperprolactinaemia   56
    male   48, 194, 198–201, 202, 232
        growth   48, *50*, 186
        treatment   175, 200–1
    post-menopausal women   207
    primary   177, 199
    secondary   199
Hypokalaemia   98, 99, 100, 102, 107
Hyponatraemia   33, 91
Hypoparathyroidism   222, 224–5
    treatment   226
Hypophosphataemia   183
Hypopituitarism   29, 44–51, 108, 179
    biochemical assessment   57, *58*
    idiopathic, of elderly   29
    and radiotherapy   58–9
Hypospadias   179
Hypotension, postural   119
Hypothalamic dysfunction   28–9
    anorexia nervosa   28, 51, 172
Hypothalamic tumours   27–8
Hypothalamus   25–33
    control of feeding   169
    diseases   27–33
    hormone deficiency   29–31, 189
    hormone excess   32–3
    hormones   25–75
Hypothyroidism (myxoedema)   75–8
    autoimmune   65–7
    causes   29, 46, 67, 76
    clinical features   76–7, 168, 189, 190
    congenital   75, 76–7
    diagnosis   63–5, 77
    hypercholesterolaemia   159, 160
    iatrogenic   76, 77
    in pregnancy   75
    prognosis   78
    treatment   77–8

IAPP *see* Islet amyloid polypeptide
IDL *see* Intermediate density lipoproteins
IGF *see* Insulin-like growth factor
IGT *see* Glucose tolerane, impaired
Immune system, pregnancy   218
Impotence   196–8
    assessment   197
    causes   196–7
    diabetes   141–2, 146, 147
    treatment   198

Infections, susceptibility in diabetes 147
Infertility
    female 50–1, 190, 210, 211, 214–16
        causes 214–15
        management 215–16
    iatrogenic 108
    male 50, *51*, 190, 200
Inhibin 40, 194, 204–5, 206
Inositol triphosphate (IP$_3$) 23, 152
Insemination, artificial (AI) 50, 200, 215
Insulin 109, *110*, 111–13
    fat metabolism and 156, 166
    growth and 180
    receptors 5, *6*, 112
    regimens 133–5
    resistance 167, 210
    secretion 3, 112
    species 133, *134*
    synthesis 3, *4*
    treatment *127*, 133–7
    types *134*
    see also Diabetes mellitus; Hyperinsulinaemia
Insulin-like growth factor 1 (IGF$_1$) 21
    female sexual function and 205, 206, 207
    growth hormone and 54, 180, 181, *182*, 187
Insulin-like growth factor 1 binding protein
        (IGF$_1$-BP) 21, *205*, 206, 207
Insulin-like growth factor 2 (IGF$_2$) 116, 180, *182*
Insulin-like growth factors (IGFs) 21, *37*, 38, 41,
        204–5
    growth and 180, 181, *182*
    polycystic ovary syndrome 210
Insulinoma 114, 115
Insulin tolerance test (hypoglycaemia stress
        test) *45*, 52, 98, 184
Interferon-γ 21
Interleukins 21
Intermediate density lipoproteins (IDL) *153*, 154,
        155, *156*
Internal carotid artery aneurysms 42
Intersex states 176–9
    management 179
Interstitial (Leydig) cells 193, 194
Intracavernosal injections 142, 197, 198
Intracranial disease, precocious puberty 191, 192
Intracranial tumours 28
In vitro fertilization 200, 215
Iodine
    deficiency 60, 67, 76–7
    metabolism 60
    radioactive, therapy 69, 73, 76, 77
    radiolabelled, thyroid uptake 65
    therapy (Lugol's iodine) 73
Iodocholesterol adrenal isotope scan 100
Iodothyronines 10–13
IP$_3$ see Inositol triphosphate
Ischaemia
    critical 149
    diabetes mellitus 139
    foot 140, 147–8
Ischaemic heart disease see Coronary heart disease
Islet amyloid polypeptide (IAPP, amylin) 125, 221
Isotope scans
    iodocholesterol adrenal 100
    Meta-iodobenzylguanidine 105
    thyroid disease 65, 68

Jaw wiring 172
Jejunoileal bypass 171–2
Jet lag 10
Joints, diabetes mellitus *138*, 142–3

Kallikreins 86–7, 116
Kallman's syndrome 29, 189, 190
Ketoacidosis, diabetic 113, 123, 127, 135
Ketoconazole *90*, 100
Ketones 113, 123, 126
Kidney 79
    adrenal cortex interactions 79, *85*
    hormones and 85–8
Kinins 86–7, 88, 117–18
Klinefelter's syndrome 177, 190

Lactation 38–9
Lactic acidosis, diabetes 128, 132
Laron-type dwarfism 184
Laser photocoagulation, diabetic retinopathy 144
Lawrence–Moon–Biedl syndrome 168
LCAT see Lecithin-cholesterol acyltransferase
LDL see Low-density lipoproteins
Lecithin-cholesterol acyltransferase (LCAT) *153*,
        154, 156
Legs, restless 145
Leucine enkephalin 80
Leucocytes
    function in diabetes *138*, 147, *148*
    hormone receptors 21
Leukotrienes 17, *18*, 19
Leydig-cell tumours 201
Leydig (interstitial) cells 193, 194
LH see Luteinizing hormone
LHRH see Luteinizing hormone-releasing hormone
Libido 175, 195, 207
Light
    pineal gland responses 10
    ultraviolet (UV) 13, 222
Light–dark rhythms 19
Liothyronine 46, 77–8
Lipid-lowering drugs 163–5
Lipids 151–4
Lipoprotein lipase (LPL) 155, 156, 157
    deficiency 160
Lipoproteins 151, 154–61
    abnormalities of metabolism 160–1
    constitution *156*
    electrophoretic mobility *160*
    factors affecting metabolism 156–9
β-Lipotrophin (β-LPH) 36
Liver disease
    diabetes mellitus *138*, 142
    hyperlipoproteinaemia 159
    osteomalacia 223
Low-density lipoprotein (LDL) receptors 155
    inherited deficiency 156, 160
Low-density lipoproteins (LDL) *153*, 154, 155,
        156
    factors affecting 157, 158, 159
Low-T$_3$ syndrome *13*, 63, 77
β-LPH see β-Lipotrophin
LPL see Lipoprotein lipase
Lugol's iodine 73

Lung carcinoma
  Antidiuretic hormone-secreting   33, 108
  gynaecomastia   202
  small-cell   96, 107, *117*
Luteal phase, short   214, 215
Luteinizing hormone (LH)   39–41, 197
  deficiency   44, 47–51, *58*, 200, 213
  gonadal failure   190
  male hypogonadism   199
  male sexual development and   179, 194
  menopausal women   207
  mid-cycle surge   206–7
  polycystic ovary syndrome   210
  puberty   187
  secretion   3, 26, 33, *34*, 40–1
  structure   3, *5*, 39
  tumours secreting   41
Luteinizing hormone-releasing hormone (LHRH) *see*
      Gonadotrophin-releasing hormone
Lymphoma, thyroid   68–9
Lysyl-bradykinin   86

McCune–Albright syndrome   191, 231
Macroadenomas, pituitary   41
Macroprolactinoma   55
Macrosomia   125
Maculopathy, diabetic   143–4
Magnesium   219
Magnetic resonance imaging (MRI)   105
Males
  infertility   50, *51*, 190, 200
  luteinizing hormone and follicle-stimulating
      hormone deficiency   48–50
  sexual differentiation   173–5
  sexual function   193–203
Malignancy   107–8
  consequences of treatment   108
  hypercalcaemia of   107, 230
  see also Tumours
MAO *see* Monoamine oxidase
Medroxyprogesterone acetate   192, 211
Melanocyte-stimulating hormones (α-MSH and
      β-MSH)   36
Melatonin   9–10
Menarche   187
Meningiomas   28, 107
Meningitis   28
Menopausal gonadotrophin, human (HMG)   50, *51*,
      216
Menopause (climacteric)   41, 207, 214
  hormone replacement therapy   208
  hot flushes   41, 118, 207
  male   194
MEN *see* Multiple endocrine neoplasia syndromes
Menorrhagia   214
Menstrual cycle   19, 40, 206–7
Menstruation, irregular   210
Messenger RNA (mRNA)   1, *2*
Mesterolone   200
Metabolic rate, obesity   167–8
Meta-iodobenzylbenzylguanidine (MIBG) scans   105
Metastases
  bone   230
  pituitary   41–2
  thyroid   69

Metformin   128, 132, 133
Methionine enkephalin (met-enkephalin)   36, 80
α-Methylparatyrosine   105
Metyrapone   53, *90*, 100
Microadenomas, pituitary   41
Microalbuminuria   141, 149
Micropenis   179
Microprolactinoma   55
MIF *see* Mullerian inhibitory factor
Mineralocorticoids   79, 80, 82–3
  control of secretion   84
  synthesis   16
  see also Aldosterone
Mithramycin   230, 233
MIT *see* Monoiodotyrosine
Mitotane (opDDD)   53, *90*, 100
Monoamine oxidase (MAO)   9
Monoamines   6–10
  phenylalanine derivatives   6–9
  tryptophan derivatives   9–10
Monocytes, vitamin D receptors   15
Monoiodotyrosine (MIT)   *11*, 12, 62
Mononeuropathies, diabetes mellitus   146
Motilin   *100*, 111
Motor neuropathy, diabetes mellitus   145, 147, *148*
MRI *see* Magnetic resonance imaging
mRNA *see* Messenger RNA
MSH *see* Melanocyte-stimulating hormones
Mullerian ducts   174, *175*, 204
Mullerian inhibitory factor (MIF)   *173*, 174, *176*,
      177
Multiple endocrine neoplasia (MEN) syndromes   69,
      105
Myasthenia gravis   120
Myeloma   230
Myocardial infarction   140
Myxoedema
  coma   77–8
  'madness'   75, 78
  pretibial   66, 71
  see also Hypothyroidism

Necrobiosis lipoidica diabeticorum   142
Negative feedback inhibition   20–1
Nelson's syndrome   53, 98, 99
Neonates, thyrotoxicosis   75
Nephroblastoma   103
Nephrotic syndrome   159
Nesidioblastosis   114, 115
Neuroblastoma   104
Neurofibromas   105
Neuroglycopenia   115
Neuropathic foot   147
Neuropathies, diabetic   *138*, 141, 142, 144–7
Neuropeptide Y (NPY)   29, 111, 169
Neurophysins   26
Neurotensin   109
Nicotinic acid and derivatives   164
Nocturia   30
Noradrenaline (norepinephrine)   6–9, 80, 84
NPY *see* Neuropeptide Y

OAF *see* Osteoclast-activating factors
Obesity   165–72

complicating other conditions 168–9
Cushing's syndrome 97, 98, 168–9
effects 165
hyperlipidaemia 157, 160, 164
management 169–72
pathogenesis 29, 165–9
polycystic ovary syndrome 168, 210, 211
type II diabetes 125, 168
Oedema
ankle 98
pulmonary 140
Oestradiol (E$_2$) *16*, 192, 204, 205
menstrual cycle 206, 207
Oestrogens
adrenal 83
excess 83, 202
gonadotrophin secretion and 40
growth and 187
hypertensive effects 89
lipoprotein metabolism and 157, 158
polycystic ovary syndrome 210
post-menopausal women 207
replacement therapy (HRT) 50, 158, 208, 209, 232
synthesis *16*
treatment 48, 212–13
tumours secreting 201, 202, 203
Oligomenorrhoea 28, 213–14
Oligospermia 198, *199*, 200
Onycholysis 71
OpDDD *see* Mitotane
Ophthalmoplegia, external 43, 146
Optic chiasm, pituitary tumours damaging 42–3
Oral contraceptives
hyperlipidaemia and 158, 161, 164
hypertension and 89
post-pill amenorrhoea 213
treatment 190, 213
weight gain 169
Oral hypoglycaemic agents 131–3
Orchidopexy 180
Osmolality, plasma/urine 30–1, 33
Osteoarthritis, diabetes mellitus 143
Osteoblasts 230–1
Osteoclast-activating factors (OAF) 107, 230
Osteoclastomas (brown tumours) *228*
Osteoclasts 15, 231
Osteocytes 231
Osteodystrophy, renal 102, 224, 229
Osteomalacia 221–6
biochemical changes 223
histological and radiological features 223
treatment 226
Osteomyelitis, diabetes 149
Osteopenia *228*
Osteoporosis 56, 98, 207, 231–2
Ovarian agenesis 209
Ovarian failure
menopausal 207
premature 208
Ovarian neoplasia 209
Ovaries 204–8
anatomy 204–6
development 173–4, 204
disease and dysfunction 209–14
resistant ovary syndrome 208

ultrasound 189, 210–11
Overweight 133, 165
Ovulation 41, 207
induction 216
Ovum, fertilized 217
Oxandrolone 189–90
Oxytocin 26–7

Paget's disease of bone 221, 233
Pain sensation 18
Pamidronate 230, 233
Pancreatic carcinoma 126
Pancreatic diseases, diabetes 125–6
Pancreatic endocrine tumours 113–14
Pancreatic polypeptide (PP) *110*, 111
Pancreatitis 125, 222
Panhypopituitarism 28
Papaverine 142, 197, 198
Papilloedema 224
Paracrine actions 1, 109
Paraesthesiae, hypocalcaemia 224
Parathyroid adenoma 228
Parathyroid carcinoma 228
Parathyroid glands 221
Parathyroid hormone (PTH) 15, *219*, 220, 221
deficiency 222, 224–5
excess *see* Hyperparathyroidism
serum 223
tissue resistance 225
Parathyroid hormone (PTH)-related peptide (PTHrp) 107, 230
Parathyroid hyperplasia 228
Parturition 18
PDGF *see* Platelet-derived growth factor
Pendred's syndrome 68
Penile implants 198
Pen injectors, insulin 135
Penis
erectile function 195–8
small 201
Pepperpot skull 228
Peptidases 6
Peptide hormones 1–6
clearance 6
secondary structure 3, 5
secretion 3–4
synthesis 1–3, *4*
target cell interaction 5–6, 22–3
transport 5
Peptide YY 111
Perchlorate discharge test 65, 68
Peripheral vascular disease, diabetes *138*, 140, 141
Peritoneal dialysis 230
PGI$_2$ *see* Prostacyclin
Phaeochromocytoma 89, 104–5, 119
Phenoxybenzamine 105
Phenylethanolamine-*N*-methyltransferase 7, 79
Phosphate *219*
oral treatment 230
serum 223, 227, 228
urinary 227
Phosphatidyl inositol derivatives 23, *24*
Phospholipids 152
Photocoagulation therapy, diabetic retinopathy 144
Phytates, dietary 222

Pigmentation 37
  Addison's disease 91, 94
  Cushing's disease 52, 98, 107
  geographical 191, 231
  Nelson's syndrome 53
Pineal gland 9–10
Pituitary 25
  anatomical relations 35–6
  anterior 33–58
    control of hormone secretion 26, 35
    diseases 41–58, 189
    hormones 33, 34, 36–41
  blood supply 34–5
  innervation 35
  posterior 25, 26–7
Pituitary apoplexy 42
Pituitary tumours 41, 42–58, 199
  adrenocorticotrophic hormone-secreting 41,
    51–3, 96, 99
  assessment 57, 58
  diabetes insipidus 30, 42, 44
  effects 42–57
  growth hormone secreting 41, 53–5, 57, 187
  hormone deficiency and 45–52
  macroadenoma 42
  microadenoma 42
  prolactin-secreting 56–7
  structural effects 28, 35–6, 42–4
  treatment 53, 55, 57–8, 99
Placental hormones 217
Placental lactogen, human (HPL) 217
Plastic surgery see Cosmetic surgrey
Platelet-derived growth factor (PDGF) 162
Platelets 18–19
Plicamycin 230, 233
Polycystic ovary syndrome 141, 209–11, 210,
    213
  hirsutism 210, 211, 212
  obesity 168, 210, 211
Polydipsia, primary 30, 31
Polyol pathway 139
Polyuria 30
POMC see Pro-opiomelanocortin
Post-coital test 215
Post-partum amenorrhoea 213
Post-partum depression 218
Post-partum thyroiditis 67, 76, 218
Postural hypotension 119
Potassium
  Conn's syndrome 99
  in differential diagnosis of Cushing's
    syndrome 98
  therapy in ketoacidosis 127
PP see Pancreatic polypeptide
Prader orchidometer 48
Prader–Willi syndrome 168
Prealbumin, thyroid hormone binding 12–13, 63
Prednisolone 93, 211, 216
Pregnancy
  diabetes in 125
  endocrinology 216–18
  hypertension 89
  lipoprotein metabolism 157
  thyroid function 63, 67, 74–5, 217–18
Pregnanetriol, urinary 95
Premenstrual syndrome 213

Prenatal diagnosis, congenital adrenal
    hypeplasia 94, 95
Preprohormones 2, 3
Priapism 198
Primoteston (mixed testosterone esters) 48–50,
    185, 189, 190, 201
Probucol 165
Progesterone 192, 205, 206, 207, 216–17
  anovulatory cycles 214
  receptors 107
  synthesis 16
Progestogens 158, 192, 211, 212
Proglucagon 111
Prohormones 2, 3
Proinsulin 4
Prolactin 38–9, 197
  deficiency 28, 51
  excess see Hyperprolactinaemia
  pregnancy 217
  secretion 3–4, 33, 34, 38
Prolactin-inhibitory factor (dopamine) 19, 26, 38
Prolactinomas 41, 55–6, 57
Prolactin-releasing factors 38
Pro-opiomelanocortin (POMC) 36
Propranolol 74, 105
Propylthiouracil (PTU) 72–3, 74, 75
Prostacyclin (PGI$_2$) 17, 18
Prostaglandins 17–19, 87
Prostate, tumours of 107
Protein, dietary intake 157
Protein hormones see Peptide hormones
Proteinuria, diabetes 149
Proton pump inhibitors 114
Pruritus vulvae 122
Pseudo-Cushing's syndrome, alcohol-induced 96–7
Pseudohermaphroditism
  female 176–7, 178
  male 176, 177, 178–9
Pseudohypoparathyroidism 225–6
Pseudopseudohypoparathyroidism 225–6
Pseudopuberty, precocious 83, 191
Pseudotabes, diabetes mellitus 147
Psychiatric disorders
  Cushing's syndrome 97
  hypothyroidism 75, 78
Psychosocial problems
  diabetes mellitus 137
  impotence 197
  precocious puberty 192
Psychotherapy, anorexia nervosa 172
PTH see Parathyroid hormone
PTHrp see Parathyroid hormone-related peptide
PTU see Propylthiouracil
Puberty 39, 187–92, 194
  delayed 28, 48, 187–91
  growth spurt 181, 182, 183, 187
  gynaecomastia 187, 194, 202
  precocious 186, 191–2
Pulmonary oedema 140

Quettelet index, BMI 165

Race
  hirsutism and 212

lipoprotein metabolism and   157
management of diabetes and   130–1
osteoporosis and   232
Paget's disease and   233
Radiculopathy, truncal   146
Radiotherapy   58, 108
Receptors
    arachidonic acid derivatives   17
    down-regulation   5–6, 22
    induction   22
    monoamine   8
    peptide hormones   5, *6*
    steroid hormones   15
5α-Reductase   *177*, 178, 211
    deficiency   179
Reifenstein's syndrome   175, 178
Relaxin   206
Release-inhibiting factors   19–20
Releasing factors   19
Renal adenocarcinoma   103, 108
Renal disease
    diabetes mellitus   *138*, 140–1
    endocrine manifestations   101–3
    hyperlipidaemia   159, 160, 161
Renal failure   89, 101–2
    hypocalcaemia and osteomalacia   222, 224
    vitamin D supplements   226
Renal osteodystrophy   102, 224, 229
Renal tubular disorders   102–3
Renal tumours   103
Renin   21, 85–6, *87*, 91
    deficiency   *90*
    tumours secreting   *101*, 103
Renin–angiotensin system   84, 85–6, 88
Renovascular hypertension   89, 102
Resistant ovary syndrome   208
Restandol (mixed testosterone esters)   200
Restless legs   145
Retinopathy, diabetic   141, 143–4
Retroperitoneal tumours (sarcomas)   115, 116
Rhythms, hormone secretion   19
Ribosomes   1–3
Rickets   180, 223
    renal   102
    vitamin D-resistant   183
Romberg's sign, positive   147
Rugger-jersey spine   224, 229

Salt balance   *87*, 88
Sarcoidosis   15, 28
Satiety, CNS control   169
Schmidt's syndrome   92
Screening, complications in diabetes   149–50
Seasonal breeding   10
Second messengers   22–4
Secretin   109, *110*
Semen analysis   215
Seminomas, testicular   201
Sensory neuropathy, diabetes mellitus   144–5, 147, *148*
Serotonin (5-hydroxytryptamine)   9–10, 114, 117–18
Sertoli cells   *193*, 194
Sertoli cell tumours   202
Sex

behavioural   174–5
chromosomal   173
gonadal   173–4
heart disease risk and   163
lipoprotein metabolism and   156–7
osteoporosis and   232
phenotypic   174, *175*, *176*
Sex-cord tumours, testicular   201
Sex hormone-binding globulin (SHBG)   15, 210, 212, 213
Sex steroids   15–17
    adrenal   83–4
    gonadotrophin secretion and   40
    growth and   180–1, 185, 187
    synthesis   *16*
    see also Androgens; Oestrogens
Sexual development
    abnormalities   176–9
    Tanner staging   187, *188*
Sexual differentiation   173–5
Sexual function
    female   204–18
    male   193–203
Sexual phenotype, unsatisfactory   201
SHBG *see* Sex hormone-binding globulin
Sheehan's syndrome   42, 51
Short luteal phase   214, 215
Shoulder, frozen   143
Sipple syndrome   105
Skin disease, diabetes mellitus   *138*, 142
Skin pigmentation *see* Pigmentation
Sleep, growth hormone secretion   181, *183*, 185
Small stature   28, 182–6, 190
    causes   183–4
    clinical features   184
    familial/constitutional   183, 186
    investigations   47, 184–5
    treatment   185–6
Smoking
    heart disease risk and   163
    lipoprotein metabolism and   157, 164
Social deprivation, childhood   183, 184
Sodium deficiency   33
Sodium fluoride (NaF)   232
Somatomedins *see* Insulin-like growth factors
Somatostatin   20, 84
    analogue treatment   55, 57, 113
    gut-derived   109, *110*, 111
    hypothalamic   26, 38, 39
Somatostatinoma   114, 126
Sorbitol   139, 144
Spermatogenesis   41
    onset   187, 194
    reduced   48, 198
Sperm invasion test   215
Spinal cord, diabetes mellitus   147
Spironolactone   100–1, 196, 213
Starvation   51, 115, 213
Stature
    eunuchoid   48, *49*, 54, 177, 186, 199
    small   28, 47, 182–6, 190
    tall   186–7
Sterility, iatrogenic   108
Steroids   4, 13–17
    anabolic   189–90, 212
    see also Corticosteroids; Sex steroids; Vitamin D

Streptozotocin 113, 114
Stress 84
Striae 97, 169
Stroke 140
Subperiosteal erosions *228*
Sudden death 146
Sulphatase, placental 217
Sulphonylurea drugs 115, 131–2
Sunlight exposure 13, 222
Sustanon (mixed testosterone esters) 48–50, 185, 189, 190, 201
Sweating
  gustatory 119, 146
  unexplained 119
Sympathetic nervous system 84, 88
Synacthen test, short *45*, 91–2

T_3 *see* Triiodothyronine
T_4 *see* Thyroxine
Tanner charts 187, *188*
TBG *see* Thyroid-binding globulin
Technetium, radiolabelled 65
Tendon xanthomata 161
Teratomas 108, 201
Testes 193–4
  anatomy *193*, 194
  development 173–4, 193–4
  hormonal control 194, *195*
  incomplete descent 179–80
  maldescent (ectopic) 179–80
  removal of abnormal 179
  size assessment 48
Testicular tumours 201–2
Testosterone *16*, 17, 21, 83, 204
  congenital adrenal hyperplasia 94
  control of secretion 41
  deficiency 48, 199, 200–1
  growth and 187
  hirsutism and 212
  ovarian tumours secreting 209
  penile erection and 195–6, 197
  polycystic ovary syndrome 210
  precocious puberty 191, 192
  resistance 178
  sexual development and 174–5, *176, 177*, 194
  treatment 48–50, 185, 189, 190, 200–1
Tetany 224
Tetracosactrin (Synacthen), test, short *46*, 91–2
Theca cells 204
Thermogenin 167
Thiazide diuretics
  adverse effects 114, 125, 158, 161, 196
  treatment 229
Thromboxane (TXA_2) 17, 18–19
Thymomas 120
Thymosins 120
Thymus 120
  congenital agenesis 120
  hormones 120
Thyroglobulin 10–11, 62
Thyroid adenomas
  benign non-toxic 68
  toxic ('hot nodule') 65, 68, *70*
Thyroid antibodies 65, 66, 74, 77

Thyroid antimicrosomal antibodies 65, 66, 67, 74, 77, 218
Thyroid-binding globulin (TBG) 12–13, 63, 217
Thyroid bruit 71
Thyroid carcinoma
  anaplastic 69
  follicular 69
  medullary 69, 105–6
  papillary 69
Thyroidectomy
  partial 73, 76, 77
  total 69
Thyroid eye disease 66, 70–1, *72*
Thyroid function tests 63–5, 71, 77, 190
  pregnancy 74, 217–18
Thyroid gland 60–78
  anatomy 60–2
  autoimmune disease 65–7
  C-cells (parafollicular cells) 221
  diseases 67–78
  histology 10–11, 62
  irradiation 108
Thyroid hormones 4, 10–13, 62–7
  in blood 12–13, 63–5
  control of secretion 62–3
  patterns of release 12
  synthesis 11–12, 60, 62
  target cell interactions 13
  see also Thyroxine; Triiodothyronine
Thyroiditis 65
  Hashimoto's *see* Hashimoto's thyroiditis
  post-partum 67, 76, 218
  subacute 67, 76
Thyroid lymphoma 68–9
Thyroid-stimulating hormone (TSH) 12, 39, 62
  adrenocortical failure 91, 92
  deficiency 46, 47, 57, *58*
  in pregnancy 63, 74, 217–18
  secretion 26, 33, *34*, 39, 62
  structure 3, *5*
  thyroid disease 64, 71, 77, *78*
  tumours secreting 41
Thyroid-stimulating immunoglobulins (TSI) 65, *66*, 75
Thyroid storm 73–4
Thyroid tumours 65, 68–9
Thyrotoxicosis 69–74
  causes 68, *69*, *70*
  clinical features 70–1, 119, 186, 202, 213, 232
  diagnosis 63–5, 71
  hyperemesis gravidarum and 75, 218
  iatrogenic or factitious *70*, 71
  neonates 75
  in pregnancy 74–5
  prognosis 73
  thyroid storm 73–4
  treatment 71–3, 76, 77
  see also Graves' disease
Thyrotrophin-releasing hormone (TRH) 26, 39, 62
  deficiency *29*
  test *46, 47, 58*
Thyroxine (T_4) 10–13, 62–7
  adrenocortical failure 91, 92
  in blood 12–13, 63–5
  control of secretion 62–3
  replacement therapy 46, 57, 75, 77

serum concentrations   46, 63, *64*, 71, 77, 78
   synthesis   11–12, 60, 62
   target cell interactions   13
Tolbutamide   132, 133
Tooth sockets, loss of lamina dura   228
Transfer RNA (tRNA)   3
Transfrontal surgery, pituitary tumours   58
Transsphenoidal surgery, pituitary tumours   58
Transthyretin (prealbumin)   12–13, 63
Trauma, hypothalamic dysfunction   28
TRH *see* Thyrotrophin-releasing hormone
Triglycerides   151, 152
   serum
      factors affecting   156–7, 158
      heart disease risk and   163
Triiodothyronine (T$_3$)   10–13, 62–7
   in blood   12–13, 63–5
   control of secretion   62–3
   fat metabolism and   167
   reverse (rT$_3$)   *12*, 13, 63
   serum concentrations   46, 64, 71, 77, *78*
   synthesis   11–12, 60, 62
   target cell interacitons   13
   therapy   46, 77–8
   toxicosis   71
tRNA *see* Transfer RNA
Trophoblastic tumours   75, 108
Trousseau's test   224
Tryptophan   116
TSH *see* Thyroid-stimulating hormone
TSI *see* Thyroid-stimulating immunoglobulins
Tuberculosis   28, 90, 92
Tumour necrosis factors   21
Tumours
   ectopic hormone secretion   107
   hormone dependence   107
   hormone production   108
   see also Malignancy
Turner's syndrome   177–8, 184, 190, 209
   male   178
TXA$_2$ *see* Thromboxane
Tyrosine hydroxylase   7

Ulcers
   heel   149
   neuropathic   147
Ultrasound
   ovarian   189, 210–11
   thyroid gland   65, 68
Ultraviolet (UV) light   13, 222

Vagal denervation of heart   146
Vanillyl mandelic acid (VMA)   *9*
Vascular disease
   diabetes   140, 141, 142
   pituitary   42
Vascular malformations   28
Vasoactive intestinal polypeptide (VIP)   109, 110–11, 113, 196
Vasodilator drugs   119
Ventromedial nucleus (VMN) of hypothalamus   169

Very low-density lipoproteins (VLDL)   151, 154, 155, *156*
   factors affecting   157, 158, 159
   metabolism   152, *153*
Vipomas   113
VIP *see* Vasoactive intestinal polypeptide
Virilization   83, 178, 211
   congenital adrenal hyperplasia   93, 94, 95
Virus infections, diabetes and   124
Visual acuity, hyperglycaemia and   122
Visual field defects   42, *43*
Vitamin D   13–15, 102, 220
   deficiency   222–3
   dietary   14
   endogenous   14
   metabolism   *14*, 15
   supplements   14–15, 102, 226
   target cell interactions   15
   tissue resistance   223
Vitamin D$_2$ (ergocalciferol)   14–15, 220, 226
Vitamin D$_3$ (cholecalciferol)   14, 220
Vitamin D-binding protein (DBP)   15
Vitamin D-resistant rickets   183
Vitrectomy   144
VLDL *see* Very low-density lipoproteins
VMA *see* Vanillyl mandelic acid
VMN *see* Ventromedial nucleus
Von Hippel–Lindau syndrome   103, 105
Von Recklinghausen's disease   105

Water balance   *87*, 88
Water deprivation test   *31*
Waterhouse–Friderichsen syndrome   92
Water restriction   33
Weight gain, drug-induced   169
Weight loss
   amenorrhoea and oligomenorrhoea   213
   diabetes mellitus   131, 133, 150
   hyperlipoproteinaemia   164
   obesity   169–72
Wermer's syndrome   105
White blood cells *see* Leucocytes
Wilms' tumour   103
Wolffian ducts   174, *175*

Xanthelasmata   161
Xanthomata
   eruptive   161
   tendon   161
XO syndrome (Turner's)   177–8, 184, 190, 209
XX males   174, 177
XXY syndrome (Klinefelter's)   177, 190
XY females   177
XYY syndrome   177

Y chromosome   173, 174
Yolk-sac tumours, testicular   201
Yttrium implants, pituitary tumours   59

Zollinger–Ellison syndrome   105, 114